D0470246

EMERGENCY
SERVICES STRESS

EMERGENCY SERVICES STRESS

Guidelines for Preserving the Health and Careers of Emergency Services Personnel

JEFFREY T. MITCHELL, Ph.D.
GRADY P. BRAY, Ph.D.

Continuing Education Series
Richard L. Judd, Ph.D., Series Editor

A BRADY BOOK
PRENTICE HALL BUILDING
Englewood Cliffs, New Jersey 07632

Library of Congress Cataloging-in-Publication Data

Mitchell, Jeffrey T.
    Emergency services stress : guidelines for preserving the health
and careers of emergency services personnel / Jeffrey T. Mitchell,
Grady P. Bray.
        p.   cm. -- (Continuing education series)
    "A Brady book."
    Bibliography: p.
    Includes index.
    ISBN 0-89303-687-0
    1. Emergency medical personnel--Mental health--United States.
2. Emergency medical personnel--United States--Job stress.
3. Stress management.   I. Bray, Grady P.   II. Title.   III. Series:
Continuing education series (Englewood Cliffs, N.J.)
RA645.5.M57   1990
362.1'8'019--dc20   89-8596
                                                                CIP

Editorial/production supervision
    and interior design: *Claudia Citarella*
Cover design: *Ben Santora*
Manufacturing buyer: *David Dickey*

Printed in the United States of America

10 9 8 7 6 5 4 3 2

ISBN   0-89303-687-0

Prentice-Hall International (UK) Limited, *London*
Prentice-Hall of Australia Pty. Limited, *Sydney*
Prentice-Hall Canada Inc., *Toronto*
Prentice-Hall Hispanoamericana, S.A., *Mexico*
Prentice-Hall of India Private Limited, *New Delhi*
Prentice-Hall of Japan, Inc., *Tokyo*
Simon & Schuster Asia Pte. Ltd., *Singapore*
Editora Prentice-Hall do Brasil, Ltda., *Rio de Janeiro*

To all emergency services personnel who have given so much, so generously, and to whom we owe so much. Thank you.

CONTENTS

2

EMERGENCY SERVICES STRESS   17

3

DISTRESS SIGNALS   37

4

STRESS SURVIVAL SKILLS   61

5

ORGANIZATION-SPONSORED STRESS SURVIVAL SKILLS   81

6

LIFELONG STRESS MANAGEMENT STRATEGIES   99

7

CRITICAL INCIDENT STRESS DEBRIEFING TEAM   131

8

STRESS CONTROL MODEL FOR EMERGENCY SERVICES   153

APPENDIX: STRESS MEASUREMENT SCALES   165

INDEX   179

FOREWORD

Emergency Services Stress, by Jeffrey Mitchell, Ph.D. and Grady Bray, Ph.D., inaugurates a series of works designed to serve the continuing education needs of emergency medical and other emergency personnel. As the complexities and professional requirements of emergency services increase, so does the literature of the field. Prentice Hall foresaw this need and under the leadership of Claire Merrick, this series was conceived.

The development and production of texts, periodicals, audiovisual materials, and research are important factors in the achievement of professionalism at all emergency service levels. Continuing education materials are a vital part of this growth. It is a well-recognized principle in all professions that continuing education is a mandate for maintenance and enhancement of skills and knowledge. Emergency service is no exception. A series designed to bring current and updated information on the emergency field is an important contribution.

It is appropriate that the first of this series deals with a subject that directly affects the capability of personnel to do their job competently and in an optimum manner. *Emergency Services Stress* addresses in one text— the only one currently available—the issue of stress and its impact on emergency services personnel. This work is a pathbreaker and fills a significant void.

Stress has always been with humans since our beginnings. Its recognition, management, and programs dealing with it are more recent phenomena. Recall that post-traumatic stress disorder is an entity of stress disorders classified only within the past fifteen years, mainly coming as a negative by-product of the Vietnam war. Mitchell and Bray are themselves pathbreakers in this field and have produced impressive offerings to the emergency professions.

   Emergency Services Stress provides important information on the nature of stress reduction programs, and includes an excellent section on Critical Incident Stress Debriefing (CISD). It is a significant work.

   Emergency Services Stress will be a valuable addition to the library of all emergency personnel.

Richard L. Judd, Ph.D., EMSI, NREMTA
Series Editor
Professor of Emergency Medical Sciences
Central Connecticut State University
New Britain, CT

FOREWORD

On the first page of this book, the authors almost casually present two little pieces of information that could serve as the gateway to improved health and longer lives for emergency service personnel and other people everywhere. First, they report the Surgeon General's estimate that "80 percent of the people who die of nontraumatic causes actually die of stress diseases." Then they state that life without stress is impossible.

For action-oriented people who really care about themselves and others the response to this information should be almost automatic: If stress-related diseases can kill you before your time, and if stress is an unavoidable part of living, then we must learn how to control or manage stress in ourselves and in our surroundings. Before we can control or manage anything, we must have a sound understanding of that which we seek to control—in this case, stress.

That's what this book offers—a solid understanding of stress in all its dimensions (with a street-wise emphasis on emergency care providers and their working environment)—and lots of common sense keys to the control and management of stress. Furthermore, the authors have organized and written this book for a specific audience, emergency responders. The order in which the materials are presented makes a lot of sense, graphic illustrations are used generously and appropriately, and each chapter ends with a thoughtful summary.

As a veteran speaker and writer in the emergency medical services field, I've noticed that emergency response people are always impressed by written or spoken words that accurately and simply explain the obvious—simple truths and common sense. Jeff Mitchell and Grady Bray have created an impressive book that does just that. It is impressive because it cuts through the technical mystique of psychology and human behavior. It presents simple truths and common sense in understandable, easy-to-read format. It could become a catalyst for positive personal change and growth in people who are being devoured from the inside out by the negative aspects of uncontrolled stress.

I found valuable information in every chapter; I've already implemented some of the authors' suggestions and strategies into my own personal and professional lives. At one point, they offer strategies to control stress "so that one's life becomes more balanced." In reading those materials, I thought of so many good people who give their emotional entirety to rescuing and caring for others. Theirs are lives out of balance. So often they are consumed by their passion to serve others. So often I have seen a need for a book like this one, to offer to a friend or colleague in desperate need of that elusive balance.

In another chapter, the authors make the very valid point that the simplest stress strategies tend to be the best. Again, the emphasis on common sense and simplicity sets this book apart from the writing of psychologists who have not defined and do not understand their audience. Co-author Jeff Mitchell, by contrast, in the five years prior to publishing this book, probably has had face-to-face contact with more emergency responders in North America than any other individual. The insights gathered through his travels leap from the pages of this book.

In my own travels and experience, I've noticed that very few emergency services organizations have a sufficient supply of mature, well-balanced, properly trained supervisors and managers. This book deals with that issue, emphasizing the responsibility of organizations to properly train their management staff. The authors make it clear that the bosses' "people skills" can be a major factor in employee stress.

Of course, blaming problems on the boss can lead to another form of imbalance. Specifically, the failure or refusal to accept responsibility for our personal fates or dilemmas. For some, it won't be easy to accept, but maybe the most valuable sentence in this book reads as follows: "*In order to successfully attack potentially destructive influences, emergency responders must accept primary responsibility for themselves.*"

Reading a book can be a totally forgettable experience. It depends on the book. You know a book is extraordinary when you are still "flashing back" on key concepts, phrases, or sentences days or weeks after reading it. That was my experience in reading the manuscript of this book. For example, when confronted by news of widespread abuse of drugs and alcohol,

I flashed back on the authors' description of a natural process called *exhilaration*. When I have encountered friends, associates, or employees who seem to be in an emotional holding pattern, I have flashed back on the authors' discussion of tapping internal resources to meet our full human potential.

This book has the potential for inspiring positive change in your life. From the common sense guidance on controlling stress in your personal life, to the organized concepts of Critical Incident Stress Debriefing and the "REAPER" (*R*ecognize, *E*ducate, *A*ccept, *P*ermit, *E*xplore, *R*efer) model for stress control in emergency services, the authors have molded and placed a literary cornerstone in the evolving foundation of modern emergency medical services.

James O. Page, J.D.

PREFACE

Emergency Services Stress is a product of fourteen years of stress research and teaching as well as the psychological treatment of stress conditions in emergency personnel. It is a collection of the most up-to-date concepts, strategies, and tactics which have shown success in reducing stress and enhancing the health of emergency personnel.

The material presented in this book has been shared with thousands of police officers, firefighters, emergency medical technicians, paramedics, dispatchers, nurses, disaster relief workers, and other emergency providers. In uncountable workshops and conferences, the two authors have presented the information in this book and have listened carefully to the experiences, suggestions, and ideas of emergency personnel. The valuable feedback provided by the emergency personnel enhanced the writing of the book. In a very real sense, the ideas, experiences, thoughts, suggestions, and critical reviews of emergency personnel have become a part of the book. Emergency personnel in every state and in a number of foreign countries deserve credit for sharing their thoughts with us.

No single book, no matter how well researched and written, can contain all the ideas that exist on a particular topic. That truth applies to *Emergency Services Stress* as well as it does to any other book. We hope emergency personnel will utilize this book as a starting point for the development of new policies and procedures designed to reduce stress and enhance their personal and work lives.

The authors welcome comments, ideas, criticisms, and suggestions. Whenever possible, those ideas will be incorporated into future writings.

We wish you the very best in your work. Much happiness!

ACKNOWLEDGMENTS

If writing a book is a difficult task, thanking everyone who contributed time, ideas, support, and encouragement is impossible. Authors never know where to begin and invariably forget some contributions of others. We are extremely grateful to everyone who has contributed their energies during the course of the writing of this book.

We are particularly indebted to Deborah Orandle, who typed portions of the manuscript and shared her impressions of the material. Her support helped carry the project through to completion. Thanks also go to Caroline Zimmerman and Sandy Bonadio for typing portions of the manuscript.

Vickie Harris, Lynn Kennedy-Ewing, and Dr. George Everly shared many ideas and experiences which eventually became incorporated into the book. We are grateful for their generosity in sharing their thoughts. They also constantly provided encouragement for the book and that will never be forgotten.

Critical Incident Stress Debriefing teams throughout the United States and in Canada, Norway, Germany, and Australia have been major contributors to this book by sharing their important suggestions with us during the last five years. To the leaders and members of CISD teams who have been so kind and encouraging—thank you.

A special note of thanks to Jonathan Chin, a graduate student in the Emergency Health Services Department of the University of Maryland, who worked so enthusiastically and painstakingly to arrange times for the authors to meet and write. The difficult and crowded schedules and the constantly changing priorities made his task a near-impossiblity. Yet he maintained his cheerfulness, professional attitude, and efficiency throughout the writing process.

The many priceless contributions of family members and friends as well as colleagues in both the emergency services and mental health fields made this book a reality. Whether named or unnamed, your contributions are valued and are a part of us and this book. Thank you!

With deepest appreciation,

Jeff and *Grady*

INTRODUCTION

Emergency services personnel are special in many ways. They have special personalities, special training, and special equipment. They accept challenges and expose themselves to situations that few people who work in nonemergency fields would even consider. They frequently perform extraordinary tasks that benefit the lives of their fellow human beings. Yet no matter how extraordinary they or their jobs are, emergency services personnel remain ordinary human beings. They are subject to the stresses of life and the effects of being exposed to excessive danger, destruction, and human misery.

For far too long, emergency personnel have silently endured extremes of human stress without relief. More than they would like to admit, the pressures of their jobs have had a negative impact on some of them. They have higher divorce rates than the average population. Many suffer from chronic sleep disturbance, distressing dreams, and memories. Changes in personality and increased feelings of depression, anxiety, and anger are common among these special workers. For a few, suicide has been chosen as the only way out of broken dreams and intense personal unhappiness. Healthy personnel often begin emergency work only to leave it prematurely or retire with damaged bodies and bruised minds.

The saddest thing to recognize is that the premature loss of emergency personnel or disruptions in their health and happiness is frequently preventable. If the right steps are taken early enough, significant stress reactions in emergency personnel can be prevented or lessened. Additionally, even severe stress reactions can be resolved if emergency personnel are given the right kind of immediate help by properly trained peer support personnel or mental health professionals.

Emergency Services Stress was written as a guidebook for the emergency services and individual personnel who are interested in reducing the negative aspects of stress. Its eight chapters provide the background information that is helpful in understanding stress, its causes, and its effects. They also provide a great deal of practical information that can be utilized by emergency services personnel to prevent, mitigate, or recover from the stress associated with emergency work.

The guidelines presented in this book are ideas developed on the basis of experience and research. They are not equally applicable to all emergency workers in all jurisdictions. Local policies, laws, regulations, and operating procedures should be followed whenever the guidelines in the book are in conflict with local policies and procedures.

Emergency personnel are too special to ignore. They need assistance in coping with stress if they are to remain healthy and happy in their special work. *Emergency Services Stress* is the first step in controlling stress. The next steps are up to those who read the book. We hope the book will help in making the next steps the right ones.

ABOUT THE AUTHORS

Jeffrey T. Mitchell, Ph.D. is an assistant professor of Emergency Health Services at the University of Maryland Baltimore County. He is a fire and police psychologist for Howard County, Maryland. He is a certified Emergency Medical Technician Instructor and a former firefighter-paramedic with nine and a half years of field experience. For four and a half years he served as a regional coordinator of emergency medical services for a five-county area in Maryland. Dr. Mitchell is an adjunct faculty member of the National Emergency Training Center of the Federal Emergency Management Agency and has lectured throughout the United States and in several foreign countries. He developed the Critical Incident Stress Debriefing process for emergency personnel and has trained CISD teams throughout the United States and in several countries. He has over fifty publications in the emergency field. He is the senior author of another book, *Emergency Response to Crisis*. Dr. Mitchell holds a master's degree in counseling psychology, an advanced graduate certificate in clinical psychology, and a Ph.D. in the field of human development.

Grady P. Bray, Ph.D. is a psychologist/consultant in private practice and consults on a wide variety of mental health topics and services. He is the president of his own consulting firm, Human Potentials. After receiving his Ph.D. in counseling psychology from the University of Georgia in 1972, Dr. Bray served as the Director of Research for the Georgia Department of Vocational Rehabilitation. Later he taught rehabilitation services at the University of Rochester Medical School for eight years. He has many publications in the field of rehabilitation and has recently published several articles related to stress in emergency services. He lectures frequently throughout the United States. He has trained a number of Critical Incident Stress teams. He serves as an adjunct faculty for the National Emergency Training Center of the Federal Emergency Management Agency.

1

STRESS ORIENTATION

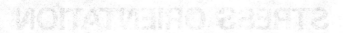

You will probably die from a stress-related disease if you are not involved in an accident. In fact, the U.S. Surgeon General has estimated that 80 percent of the people who die of nontraumatic causes actually die of stress diseases.[1] Ironically, stress is not designed by nature to kill, but rather, to enhance life. Some stress is helpful and actually essential for a full and productive life (see Figure 1–1). Positive or beneficial stress, referred to as *eustress,* is found in all forms of biological activity on earth. It helps us to be creative, productive, and to make necessary changes in our life-style that help preserve our lives and improve our happiness. Life without stress is impossible. Without stress there would be no change, growth, or productivity.[2]

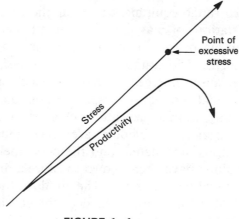

FIGURE 1–1

Most of us are more familiar with the negative aspects of stress, the painful condition we call *distress*. When stress gets out of control (distress) it becomes a destructive force that has a negative impact on our health, our personalities, our jobs, and our families.[3]

The primary purposes of this book are to provide emergency personnel with a basic understanding of stress, to encourage the productive use of positive stress (eustress), and to provide strategies and tactics of stress survival that can reduce the harmful effects of distress.

NATURE OF STRESS

The word "stress" comes directly from the ancient Latin language. It meant "force," "pressure," or "strain." Today, there are several ways to define *stress:*

- A response to a perceived threat, challenge, or change
- A physical and psychological response to any demand
- A state of psychological and physical arousal[3-7]

The common element of these definitions is that stress is a *response* to something in the environment (a "stressor"). When the environment changes, we change.

RESPONSE TO A DEMAND

An ambulance crew in quarters usually settles into a more relaxed activity level than they experience on a call. There are reports to write. They may clean and rearrange equipment and supplies, perform housekeeping tasks around the station, or play cards or watch television.

Once an alarm for a new run comes in, an obvious change occurs in the environment. The sound of the alert tones, signals, phone, or radio transmission causes emergency personnel to change their activity level radically. They quickly answer the dispatcher, put on jackets, check map books, run to the unit, unplug the battery charger, start the unit, and begin the emergency response. Their bodies are functioning at a high pitch. Muscles are tensed, pupils are dilated, and the personnel are breathing faster. The alarm tones alone have been known to cause a dramatically increased heart rate and elevated blood pressure. The minds of the crew have captured every available bit of information related to the call and they are rapidly processing it in an attempt to be prepared best for the actual work at the scene.

At this point stress is working as a positive, driving force to help the crew carry out the tasks involved with the call. As long as the stress does not become overbearing, it will continue to function as eustress—the positive type of stress.[2,3]

TYPES OF STRESS

The alarm tones in the example above represent one form of stress—an *environmental stress*. Additional environmental stressors include:[6]

- Noise
- Dirt/dust
- Overcrowding at the station
- Temperature extremes
- Clutter
- Weather conditions
- Spectators in the way
- Speed on calls
- Confined space
- Lighting
- Pressures of rapid response
- Rapid decision making
- Etc.

In addition to environmental stressors, people experience two other main types of stressors: psychosocial and personality stressors. *Psychosocial stressors* are almost anything that has to do with contact with people;[6,7] for example:

- Family relationships
- Conflicts with fellow workers
- Conflicts with the administration
- Lack of appreciation from hospital staff
- Abusive patients
- Intoxicated patients
- Media at the scene
- Etc.

Personality stressors are focused inside ourselves. They are related to the ways in which we think and feel and the memories of our past experiences.[6,7] They include:

- The inability to say "no" to someone
- The need to be liked
- Guilt feelings when we are not helping someone else
- Anxiety over our own professional competence
- A mental outlook in which we see everything as negative
- Personal sensitivity to criticism
- Extremely high expectations of ourselves
- Guilt over mistakes or not doing a perfect job
- Etc.

THE "PILEUP EFFECT"

Usually, one of these stressors alone is not sufficient to create a major stress response, but when combined, the effect can be extremely destructive. Little things have a way of piling up until they finally undermine a person's ability to cope.

The cumulative effect of small stressors can be easily equaled or surpassed by the experience of a major distressing event. These events are called *critical incidents*. More will be said about critical incidents later in the book.

THE COMFORT ZONE

Another type of stress is that caused by boredom. Lack of action, or boredom, can work against us and may be as destructive to health and happiness as too much stress.[5,8] There is a comfort zone of stress, which is a little different for each person. Too much or too little stress becomes dangerous and destructive. Everyone has to determine through experience his or her own comfort zone, to be able to avoid the harmful effects of too little or too much stress. Figure 1–2 illustrates the comfort zone and indicates that a moderate level of stress is important if a person is to maintain a high level of productivity.

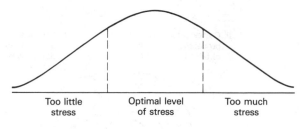

FIGURE 1–2

Generally, minor stressors produce a mild reaction, while a major stressor produces a more severe stress reaction. Later in the book you will learn how to develop a personal stress profile that will help you separate major from minor stressors. You will also learn specific strategies and techniques to help you protect yourself from distress.

PHYSICAL ASPECTS OF THE STRESS PROCESS

The stress process is an extremely complex interaction between the body and the mind. There are many intricate biochemical reactions that take place once the brain becomes aware of a stressor. Space does not permit a detailed explanation of the process. Instead, the essential features of the stress process will be summarized briefly. Although the details of the stress responses are complicated, it is important to develop an understanding of them because experience has shown that success with stress mastery strategies is much greater when the rationale for the suggested changes is understood.[9,10]

Cortex

To understand how we respond during a stress reaction, we must know the sequence of events and the changes produced during the body's response. A stress reaction begins with information entering the brain, usually through one or more of our five senses (see Figure 1–3). The information from sensory organs is gathered and processed in the cortex or outer layer of the brain. The cortex is that part of the brain which allows us to be analytical, rational, and intuitive. It contains the mechanisms for communications, creativity, conscience, problem solving, and memory. The cortex processes the

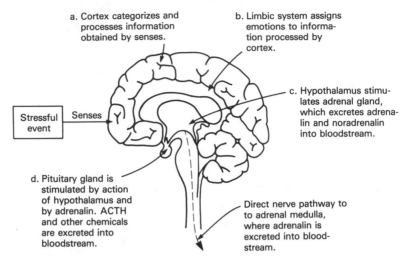

a. Cortex categorizes and processes information obtained by senses.

b. Limbic system assigns emotions to information processed by cortex.

c. Hypothalamus stimulates adrenal gland, which excretes adrenalin and noradrenalin into bloodstream.

Stressful event | Senses

d. Pituitary gland is stimulated by action of hypothalamus and by adrenalin. ACTH and other chemicals are excreted into bloodstream.

Direct nerve pathway to to adrenal medulla, where adrenalin is excreted into bloodstream.

e. Chemicals from pituitary gland stimulate adrenal cortex, which discharges additional chemicals into bloodstream. These chemicals (catecholamines) activate all other body systems.

FIGURE 1-3

information about the stressor and interprets its significance based on history (memories of previous events), logic, and predictions.

Limbic System

The information being processed by the cortex is shared with another part of the brain, called the limbic system. The limbic system has a bridging function between the more highly evolved cortex and more basic, life maintenance systems of the brain stem. In addition, the limbic system provides basic emotional "tags" such as fear, anger, love, or disgust for the information that has been passed on to it by the cortex. If the cortex and the limbic system process the information from the senses and conclude that there is a threat, challenge, or significant change to be met, a physiological stress reaction begins.[11]

Hypothalamus

Once the cortex and the limbic system have been aroused, the state of arousal is rapidly transferred to the hypothalamus. The hypothalamus is basically a communications center between the higher brain and the body. It monitors and balances a vast array of biochemical processes in the body systems. For example, it is responsible for temperature control, metabolism, and sexual excitement.

Adrenal Gland

The adrenal medulla is stimulated by messages sent down a nerve that runs directly from the hypothalamus to the inner portion of the adrenal gland (the adrenal medulla) (Figure 1-4). The adrenal medulla excretes epinephrine (adrenalin) and norepinephrine (noradrenaline) into the bloodstream when it has been stimulated by the messages sent to it by the hypothalamus.

Biochemical Response

The mere presence of epinephrine in the bloodstream influences the brain to alert the rest of the body to react to the stressor. The brain's cortex and limbic system are further aroused by the epinephrine, and very quickly, process all the information coming in through the senses. The pituitary gland is

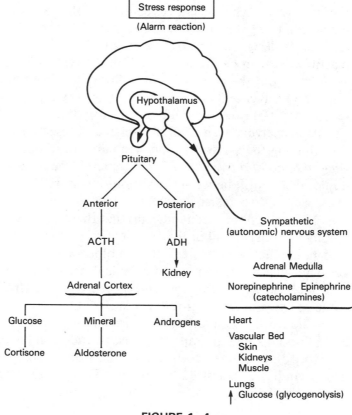

FIGURE 1-4

also stimulated to excrete a chemical called adrenocorticotropic hormone (ACTH). This chemical acts as a messenger in the bloodstream which stimulates the cortex of the adrenal gland to excrete a variety of powerful chemicals called catecholamines, which cause the entire body to prepare to deal with the stress. Muscles tighten, pupils dilate to take in more light, and the breathing rate increases, as does the heart rate and blood pressure. Cholesterol and triglyceride levels increase rapidly in the blood. Fat cells (the raw material for the liver to produce glucose, the fuel for muscles) appear in abundance. Protein (the building blocks of white blood cells and antibodies) levels in the blood increase dramatically. The liver produces ten times the amount of blood glucose than it does under nonemergency circumstances.[2]

FIGHT OR FLIGHT

The complex physiological response to stress is described as the *fight-or-flight reaction*. The hyperalert condition of the body and the mind allows the person to fight actively or to run away from the stressor. The entire stress reaction is designed for positive action. It is a healthy, normal emergency reaction that can be lifesaving. Without stress, human life would have disappeared from the earth long ago. Stress reactions give us the energy necessary to protect and defend ourselves or to withdraw when the threat is so severe that it may cost our life or seriously injure us if we continue to fight.

Hans Selye, a Canadian physician and researcher, spent his entire adult life studying the stress reaction. He named the fight-or-flight response the *general adaptation syndrome*. By "general" he means that the body organs do not distinguish between the various stressors. Joy may activate the stress response, as does fear or anxiety.[3]

More recent research indicates that there is, in fact, some distinguishing among various stimuli in the chemical responses within the body. Different catecholamines are excreted into the bloodstream for different stimuli. Anger will cause a different set of chemicals than will joy. For the purposes of this book, however, the "general" nature of the stress response has some value in explaining how stress works.[13,14]

The word "adaptation" as used in Selye's work means that the body and mind make an attempt to adjust to the stimulus or stressor. Selye uses the word "syndrome" to mean a collection of signs and symptoms which usually indicate that stress is present. The general adaptation syndrome is illustrated in Figure 1–5.[2,3]

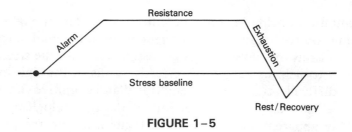

FIGURE 1-5

ALARM, RESISTANCE, AND EXHAUSTION

An alarm reaction occurs when the brain recognizes a stressful stimulus in the environment. The alarm reaction is essentially the state of psychological and physiological arousal described earlier. Once a person is aroused, he or she makes efforts to cope with the demands. Every effort, no matter how useful or effective, is part of the resistance. Resistance continues until the person is no longer capable of further resistance. Then he or she enters the exhaustion phase, in which resistance drops off and activity returns to the nonemergency state that existed before the crisis.

Rest and recovery from the stressor follows the exhaustion phase and the person is then ready for the next emergency or excitement. The General Adaptation Syndrome is activated only when an event occurs that is of an emergency nature (an unusual event which places a very high demand on one's resources). The event must exert demands that surpass the effectiveness of the more routine coping mechanisms available to the person.

PERSONAL ASPECTS OF THE STRESS RESPONSE

A stress reaction has both physical and mental elements. Remember, it is described as a state of physical and psychological arousal. In the preceding section we described the physical aspects of the stress response. Now we will pay some attention to the psychological aspects of the stress response.

The changes in emotional or cognitive function that are part of a stress response can be confusing, sometimes even frightening. Although most people can accept the outward, physical changes associated with stress, they cannot associate their absentmindedness, forgetfulness, or inability to concentrate with the stressful event they are experiencing. They place a great premium on being in control of themselves. The thought that they may be losing control because of their stress brings out denial, anger, and hostility.[15]

Just as the physical changes associated with the stress response are designed to help us cope more effectively (as in the fight-or-flight response) with difficult situations, our emotional and cognitive changes also have protective functions. But the benefits of the psychological changes are not as readily apparent since we tend to focus more on the problems associated with the signs and symptoms of the stress response instead of any of its benefits. The following section should help to shed some light on how cognitive, emotional, and behavioral reactions actually may benefit us despite their seemingly negative effects.

COGNITIVE, EMOTIONAL, AND BEHAVIORAL EFFECTS OF STRESS

As we experience increasing levels of distress, we begin to lose our mental efficiency. Our ability to remember new information begins to decrease, as does our short-term memory. We find ourselves reviewing the same material several times or asking someone to repeat the list of the items they asked us to get for them. Concentration is difficult and we become more easily distracted. Many people report a sudden flow of ideas, almost as though their minds had moved to a higher speed but without the ability to select one idea on which to focus. Our perceptions of problems change so that minor obstacles appear as major hurdles. We lose our mental flexibility and become rigid in our views of problems and solutions.[16-18]

Criticisms of our ideas or suggestions are viewed as criticisms of ourselves and we respond defensively as though we had been attacked. In essence we become a mental victim and reject the ideas, plans, or solutions suggested by others because of our singleminded endorsement of our own views.

These cognitive changes have a natural evolution or interface with the emotional changes, which can be a part of a stress response. As we become more rigid we lose our sense of humor and can no longer laugh at ourselves or the situation. Humor is one of the primary coping strategies we use to help us through traumatic events in our lives, so its loss leaves us more defenseless and vulnerable to the ravages of stress-induced emotional depletion. Another coping strategy that diminishes under stress is the ability to think clearly. The reduction in clear thinking further intensifies our vulnerability to additional stress.

The foundation for most intense personal relationships is trust. As we become distressed, our ability to trust others lessens. We fear that others will not be capable of helping us. As a result, we withdraw from the people who are our primary support and become isolated from the very people we need the most.

A vacuum is an unnatural state in physics and also in human emotions. The losses we encounter as a part of the stress reaction are replaced with increased fantasies and wishful thinking. The emotions associated with these coping strategies are personal and available only to the person developing them. To others, many of whom may be concerned and want to help, the distressed person appears more detached, alone, and not open to emotional approach. This vicious cycle is completed when the distressed person perceives friends, coworkers, and family as cold, not caring, and abandoning in their behaviors.[17]

In light of the destructiveness of these emotional and cognitive changes brought about by distress, of what possible benefit can they be? Basically, *the seemingly negative changes described above minimize the probability of emotional overload. The changes produce a psychological barrier which enables the person to function with a minimum of distracting emotional energy during a period of intense stress.* Lessening the chances of emotional overload allows a stressed person to concentrate his or her energies in the physical fight-or-flight response. *The drive for physical survival usually outweighs the emotional and cognitive drives in the person.*

The changes we have described reflect the most severe response patterns. Few people will demonstrate all of these symptoms, but familiarity with the possible changes makes one more aware of the subtle changes which indicate that a destructive distress process has started. (See Chapter 3 for a more detailed explanation of the signs and symptoms of distress.)[18-20]

SUMMARY

Stress is a state of psychological and physical arousal which comes about as a result of a threat, challenge, or change in one's environment. Stress is a normal and natural response that is designed to protect, maintain, and enhance our lives. An understanding of how stress affects us physically, mentally, and emotionally prepares us for an active emphasis on "eustress" (the positive aspects of stress) and an effective response to the negative aspects of stress ("distress").

REFERENCES

1. U.S. Surgeon General's Office. July 1988. Personal communication from Surgeon General's staff. See also Pelletier, K. R. (1977). *Mind As Healer, Mind As Slayer: A Holistic Approach to Preventing Stress Disorders.* New York: Delta Books.
2. Selye, H. (1956). *The Stress of Life.* New York: Free Press.
3. Selye, H. (1974). *Stress without Distress.* Philadelphia: J. B. Lippincott.
4. van der Kolk, B. A., Boyd, H., Krystal, J., and Greenberg, M. (1984). *Post-Traumatic Stress Disorder: Psychological and Biological Sequelae.* Washington, DC: American Psychiatric Press, 124–134.
5. Trumbull, R., and Appley, M. H. (1986). A conceptual model for the examination of stress dynamics. In M. H. Appley and R. Trumbull (Eds.). *Dynamics of Stress: Physiological, Psychological, and Social Perspectives.* New York: Plenum, 21–45.
6. Cooper, C. L. (1981). *The Stress Check.* Englewood Cliffs, NJ: Prentice-Hall.
7. Girdano, D. A., and Everly, G. S. (1986). *Controlling Stress and Tension: A Holistic Approach.* Englewood Cliffs, NJ: Prentice-Hall.
8. Frankenhaeuser, M. (1986). A psychological framework for research on human stress and coping. *Dynamics of Stress: Physiological, Psychological, and Social Perspective.* New York: Plenum, 101–116.
9. White, R. W. (1985). Strategies of adaptation: An attempt at systematic description. In A. Monat and R. S. Lazarus (Eds.), *Stress and Coping: An Anthology.* 2nd ed. New York: Columbia University Press, 121–143.
10. Everly, G. S., and Sobelman, S. A. (1987). *Assessment of the Human Stress Response.* New York: AMS Press.
11. Everly, G. S., and Rosenfeld, R. (1981). *Nature and Treatment of the Stress Response: A Practical Guide for Clinicians.* New York: Plenum.
12. Gherman, E. M. (1981). *Stress and Bottom Line: A Guide to Personal Well-Being and Corporate Health.* New York: AMACOM.
13. Cox, T. (1978). *Stress.* London: Macmillan.
14. Frankenhaeuser, M. (1975). Experimental approaches to the study of catecholamines and emotions. In L. Levi (Ed), *Emotions: Their Parameters and Measurement.* New York: Raven Press.
15. Brallier, L. (1982). *Successfully Managing Stress.* Los Altos, CA: National Nursing Review.
16. Fenz, W. D. (1964). Conflict and stress as related to physiological activation and sensory perceptual and cognitive functioning. *Psychological Monographs, 78*(8).
17. Patrick, P. K. (1981). *Health Care Worker Burnout, What It Is, What to Do about It.* Chicago: Inquiry Books.

18. Millon, T., and Everly, G. (1985). *Personality and Its Disorders.* New York: Wiley.

19. Lazarus, R., and Folkman, S. (1984). *Stress Appraisal and Coping.* New York: Springer.

20. Everly, G. S. (1989). *A Clinical Guide to the Treatment of Human Stress.* New York: Plenum.

2

EMERGENCY SERVICES STRESS

Emergency services is one of our society's most challenging and potentially rewarding vocations. Yet many who enter cannot withstand the persistent pressure of its occupational stress. There are few stressors in life that can have the destructive power associated with the stress of caring for the sick or injured. Similarly, police officers, firefighters, disaster workers, and other emergency personnel experience tremendous stress as a result of their work with and on behalf of other people. Several researchers have pointed out that the responsibility for the life and safety of others is considered a significant stressor to emergency personnel, and it may have damaging effects on their lives.[1-4]

PERSONALITY FACTORS IN EMERGENCY PERSONNEL

With the risks and demands of these professions, one has to wonder why a person would choose emergency services for a career or volunteer activity. People who choose a career with inherent powerful stressors have personalities that match them to the work or they would find it intolerable. Recent research indicates that emergency personnel, such as firefighters, paramedics, and police officers have very different personalities from the average person who has a far less risky or demanding job.[5] Emergency personnel are more interested in details than are people in most other professions. They pride themselves on a perfect job, frequently set personal standards that are extremely high, and become quite frustrated when they encounter a failure.

This attention to detail helps them to do a better job, but it also sets them up for the stress associated with a failure to achieve unusually high expectations.

Emergency personnel who are most successful usually have good internal references and are outgoing. That is, they like people and are motivated by internal factors such as the satisfaction of doing a good job. Most are somewhat less motivated by external factors such as money or promotions.[1,6]

A common trait in emergency personnel is that they are action oriented. They are quick decision makers under pressure, and task oriented. They have a difficult time postponing gratification and seek more immediate results. Most emergency personnel are easily bored. They resent false calls or abusive patients who are not truly sick because they feel that their time is being wasted. Given a choice between the scene of a disaster and just sitting around the station, they will usually choose the work.

Risk-taking behaviors accompany the action orientation in their personalities. Emergency personnel frequently expose themselves to danger as they attempt to help others. They face the serious dangers associated with exposure to disease, potentially violent people, and severely damaged automobiles and buildings with a calm and measured attitude. In their off-duty hours they frequently seek sports activities that are highly stimulating and exciting because they are easily bored and need something to keep them alert.

Emergency personnel have a very strong need to rescue or help others. This trait goes hand in hand with their action orientation and their risk taking. It is difficult for them to say "no" to any call for help which they believe is legitimate. Frustration arises when they are unable to utilize their skills to help others.

One personality factor that keeps emergency personnel on the job is their extreme sense of dedication. They keep working to help others even when it may be hurting themselves. Figure 2–1 summarizes the typical personality traits of emergency personnel.[5,7]

PATTERNS OF CHRONIC STRESS

Most people associate stress with a response to a major event. They can readily accept the impact of overwhelming emotional strain associated with massive destruction, as in an earthquake, or multiple deaths as a result of fire or motor vehicle accident. Not as clearly understood is the tremendous toll in physical, mental, and emotional resources demanded by long-term,

---

FIGURE 2-1   General Personality Traits of Emergency Personnel

Need to be in control

Obsessive (desire to do a perfect job)

Compulsive (tend to repeat the same actions for very similar events; traditional)

Highly motivated by internal factors

Action oriented

High need for stimulation

Have a need for immediate gratification

Easily bored

Risk takers

Rescue personality

Highly dedicated

Strong need to be needed

---

frequently low level stress. Stress of this type, which is often called *chronic stress* or *cumulative stress,* is often overlooked by emergency personnel attempting to correct problems they associate with stress.

Chronic stress is by its very nature deceptive. Seldom do we recognize the routine, mundane stressful issues which, after a while, feel "normal" to us. Chronic stressors are often taken for granted and few interventions are developed in response to them. Untreated, they can be as destructive as any chronic disease process.[5]

One technique that can help in the identification of chronic stressors is the development of a *stress assessment profile*. Figure 2–2 will enable you to compile a list of stressful situations that are of concern to you. The profile presents several different life components which have frequently been identified by emergency responders as sources of chronic stress. After each heading, write five specific sources of stress in your life.

FAMILY STRESSORS

Most of your family concerns have probably existed for more than three months. Few represent critical situations that will result in major life changes within the next few weeks or even months. Yet when taken as a group they can have considerable impact on the quality of your life.

FIGURE 2–2   Stress Assessment Profile: Family Stressors

Name: _____

Date: _____

Directions: List five stressors under each of the following headings. Be as specific as you can.

These things about my spouse (primary relationship) bother me:

1. _____

2. _____

3. _____

4. _____

5. _____

These things about other people in my family bother me:

1. _____

2. _____

3. _____

4. _____

5. _____

These things concern me about myself:

1. _____

2. _____

3. _____

4. _____

5. _____

These are concerns that I have about income for my family, including myself. (*Note:* It is not sufficient to say simply, ''not enough'' for this question. What do the limitations in income prevent you from doing?)

1. _____
2. _____
3. _____
4. _____
5. _____

The identification of these stressors is the beginning of a problem-solving process. Any effective approach to problem solving requires clear identification of problems so that appropriate responses can be developed.

THE PROBLEM-SOLVING PROCESS

An effective problem-solving process involves the following steps:[8]

1. Clearly identify the problem in specific terms that can be measured (i.e., how often, how many, when, what, etc.).
2. Identify possible interventions or solutions for the problem. During this phase it is important to consider all ideas that come to mind. No matter how far-fetched they may appear at first, include them in a written list of interventions.
3. Choose the intervention that seems to offer the best possible solution.
4. Implement the chosen intervention.
5. Reassess the problem to see if the strategy you selected resolved the problem.
6. If necessary, select another strategy and implement it for problem resolution.

If you select one of the problems you listed on your stress assessment profile concerning relationships with your spouse and apply the steps listed above, you should be able to develop a plan to help resolve the situation. The key to an effective plan is to break everything down into measurable components. Most situations can be broken down in this way with thought and analysis.

CONFLICT: A BASIS FOR STRESS

Most of the problems you identified may be related to conflict. Most emergency personnel have a strong need to be liked by the people around them. Conflict involves confrontation and the fear that the person with whom you are in conflict will not like you. It is often difficult to us to accept the fact that people can be angry with us and still value us as people. We struggle with the unachievable task of trying to make everyone like us, and ultimately we must fail. Not everyone is going to like us. Unless we can accept our worth and value as an inherent part of us that can never be taken away, we live with the fear that we will never do enough to deserve the love, appreciation, or respect of our friends, family, and work associates.

Conflict usually evolves out of differences in goals, values, or procedures. Unresolved conflict bothers us even though we try to block it from our minds. A much healthier approach is to discuss the differences that exist between two people and try to define the conflict from the other person's perspective. This approach is built around effective communications skills.[9]

All communications during conflict have two components: issues and affects. *Issues* are the cognitive or intellectual aspects of communications; *affects* are the emotional components of conflict. Issues and affects represent our thoughts and feelings about a conflict.

When we attempt to cope with the chronic pressure generated by conflict, we often focus on the emotions associated with the conflict rather than directing our attention and responses to the issues that constitute the problem. Increased emotional intensity produces much stronger stress responses, thus further intensifying and compounding our long-term stress.

To address this concern more accurately, we should focus our efforts and attention to the specific issue that separates us. Our emotions are not rational, nor do we choose how we feel in most situations. Rather, we experience our emotions as they evolve during life events. To focus on the emotions moves us farther from the issue we need to address.

In some situations it is helpful to reverse the roles of people involved in conflict. Each should try to summarize both the issue and the affect they think are present in the other person. Each person should have a few minutes to present his or her assessment of the other's position. Following each person's summary, the other person should give feedback concerning the accuracy of the assessment. This approach allows for an open exchange of information as well as a validity check for each person's assessment of opposing views.

Conflict is not limited to family or friends. It is also a part of the work environment. Conflict can occur with supervisors, peers, and those we supervise. Chronic stress from the work environment is as destructive as any other stressor.

The same strategies that help with family conflict can be employed to help reduce the chronic stress from the workplace. It is important to separate out these two environments because there is a tendency to release the accumulated frustrations from one area into the other. Most frequently, we find emergency personnel "dumping" the work-related stress into the confines of their home life.

This type of release is a great temptation for responders since families tend to have far fewer conditions for acceptance and love than do their employers. It is safer to scream at your spouse or children than to yell at your boss or fellow workers. Being safer does not make it more correct or appropriate; it simply transfers the tension to home rather than maintaining it in the work environment. The short-term gain is found in diluting the intensity of the frustration by spreading it over a much broader interpersonal field. However, the net effect for the stressed person is the same—tension, frustration, anger, and continued chronic stress. In situations like this the person is usually dealing only with the affect (emotion), not with the underlying issue.

CHRONIC WORK STRESSORS

One of the most consistently voiced concerns of emergency workers is shift work. Shift work is inherently stressful. It disrupts everything from biorhythms to social life. It cannot be eliminated, so emergency personnel must adjust to it. But adjustment to something does not mean that people are going to like it.

Other chronic stressors associated with work may be more difficult to define. It is easy to recognize the chronic stress from overloaded working conditions, but seldom do most responders clearly understand the stress associated with boredom. As identified earlier, emergency responders are action-oriented people who have a need to feel involved. One of the reasons for becoming a member of an emergency team is to meet a personal need for action and adventure. These characteristics are part of what has been called the *type A* person. For the type A person, inactivity is perceived as a threat against their basic need for high activity levels. Since stress was defined in part as a response to perceived threat, it follows that inactivity or boredom would result in increased chronic stress.[10] To help clarify the chronic stressors associated with work, complete Figure 2–3.

We initially seek jobs to meet our financial needs, but as we advance in our careers we seek to meet additional needs by the different jobs that we choose. Within each person are needs to achieve the goals we set for ourselves. Many of these goals were actually established for us early in our

FIGURE 2–3   Stress Assessment Profile: Work Stressors

Name: _____

Date: _____

Directions: List five stressors under each of the following headings.

These things about my supervisors and administrators bother me:

1. _____
2. _____
3. _____
4. _____
5. _____

These things about the people I work with bother me:

1. _____
2. _____
3. _____
4. _____
5. _____

These things about my work environment bother me:

1. _____
2. _____
3. _____
4. _____
5. _____

These things about my long-term career goals bother me:

1. _____
2. _____

3. _____

4. _____

5. _____

lives by our families. These goals, beliefs, and dreams from our families became a part of us. These cumulative beliefs are part of our view of ourselves as worthwhile people. When we are accomplishing what we think we should with our lives, we are more at peace with ourselves and our level of intrapersonal stress is lower.

INTRAPERSONAL STRESS

Intrapersonal stress is that stress which occurs when we are not living our lives in either the way or style that we believe should be characteristic for us. The person who believes that he or she should be working at a certain rank or income level but who is employed far below that will experience intrapersonal stress. Personal beliefs and values are conflicted with reality. The greater the distance between the ideal level at which the person believes that he or she should be functioning and the perceived level at which he or she is functioning, the greater will be the intrapersonal stress. There are two basic strategies for coping with intrapersonal stress:

1. Lower the level of the idealized aspirations.
2. Raise the level of performance to be closer to the ideal.

Realistic evaluation, frequently requiring objective, outside help, can often help identify unrealistic goals or performance levels that are beyond a person's ability. Often, the expectations of family members place a major burden on developing youngsters. As they grow into adulthood, they maintain these family myths (beliefs) as a realistic part of their self-expectations. To be freed of these burdensome expectations can go a long way toward reducing the person's chronic stress levels and enhancing his or her quality of life.

The nature of chronic stress is such that we have to be on guard for its deceptive entry into our lives. As we become more sensitive to its influence, we can recognize it for what it is and work to remove it from our lives. The alternative is to allow chronic stressors to remain as a major consideration in our lives and suffer the loss of joy, happiness, and control that go with long-term chronic stress.

CUMULATIVE STRESS

It has been popular to refer to chronic or cumulative stress as "burnout." The word *burnout* was meaningful when it was first used,[11,12] but with overuse the term has become less meaningful because it has been diluted. People started using the term in a negative way, which did not make stress a believable problem. People got the idea that when others talked about burnout, they were just making excuses to avoid work. The term became a catch-all for every type of stress problem. Burnout became an irritating term, rather than one that helped us to understand how people become exhausted and worn out by their work.

A much cleaner, clearer term is *cumulative stress*. This term implies that a person is suffering through the buildup of variety of stresses over a period of time. *Cumulative stress reactions come about as a result of a buildup of work as well as non-work-related stressors. It usually takes a long time to build up enough stress for it to show up in a cumulative stress reaction.* In most cases cumulative stress reactions do not show up for months or even years.

Cumulative stress reactions are made up of a collection of stressful events, such as critical incidents combined with home- or family-related stressors. They may also be mixed together with organizational stressors, routine stressors on the job, and leftover stressors from one's early development as a child.

Cumulative stress reactions are a combination of acute, delayed, and chronic stressors which have developed in work and nonwork areas. They are difficult to diagnose properly and to cure because they have so many interrelated features and have taken many months or years to develop.[13-15] The development of a cumulative stress reaction is often so slow and subtle that frequently it is not even noticed as it develops. Most of the time a cumulative stress reaction is so complex that it takes special help from medical and psychological professionals to resolve it. By the time it is noticed, people who have a cumulative stress reaction may be sick or have experienced marital problems, alcoholism, and other problems. Some may have undergone personality changes or may be dysfunctioning on the job. If their condition has deteriorated significantly, they need outside professional assistance to get back on track. Those who wait too long to get help jeopardize their jobs, their families, and their health.[16]

ACUTE STRESS REACTIONS

A more noticeable type of emergency stress than the chronic type is the *acute stress reaction*. These are more noticeable because they are usually dramatic, frequently overwhelmingly powerful experiences for emergency personnel. An acute stress reaction is a reaction to one or more particularly difficult emergency calls. These calls are often called *critical incidents* because they are so powerful that they can easily overcome a person's normal ability to cope with the stress of the job. Critical incidents are extraordinary events that cause extraordinary stress reactions.[17] Examples of critical incidents are:

- Death to a fellow worker in the line of duty
- Serious injury to an emergency provider in the line of duty
- Working on a person who is a relative or close friend and who is dying or in very serious condition
- Suicide involving a fellow emergency worker
- A disaster
- A very violent person who has personally threatened the emergency provider
- Almost any case with excessive media interest
- Contact with dead or severely sick or injured children
- Death to a civilian caused by emergency operations such as an accident between the civilian's car and the responding emergency vehicle

In actuality, any event can be considered a critical incident if it has the ability to distress an emergency person by overwhelming the person's usual coping ability. Some critical incidents may affect only one to two people who are involved with it. Others are so powerful that virtually every emergency person at the scene will be strongly affected by the incident.[18]

Several recent studies indicate that better than 85 percent of emergency personnel have experienced acute stress reactions after working at one or more critical incidents similar to those presented above.[17] Fortunately, the majority of emergency personnel experience only temporary stress reactions and recover within a few weeks. Others take several months to overcome fully the effects of critical incidents, and a small number (2 to 4 percent) may experience such profound effects that their jobs, families, health, and happiness are permanently impaired (see Figure 2–4). (Strategies and techniques to lessen the impact of critical incidents and to assist in the recovery process are discussed fully in Chapters 4, 5, and 6.)

Most acute stress reactions begin either at the scene or shortly thereafter. The majority of emergency personnel report that within 24 hours they

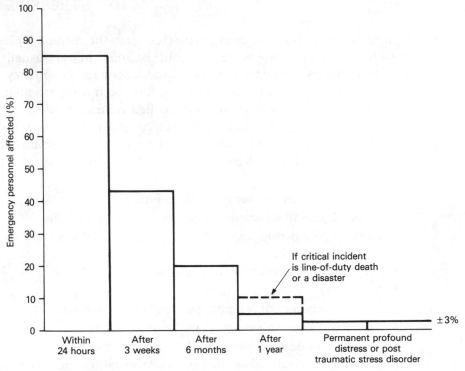

FIGURE 2–4

experience the beginning signs and symptoms of acute stress. (Chapter 3 contains an extensive discussion of the signs and symptoms of acute stress.)

DELAYED STRESS

Stress reactions do not always show up at the time of the critical incident. It is not unusual for a critical incident to have its effects days, weeks, months, and even years after it ends. Delayed stress responses are like acute stress reactions in that they are incident specific. That is, they are a direct result of a critical incident. But for a number of reasons, including, among others, the tendency of emergency medical personnel to suppress their emotions, the reactions to critical incidents are delayed.

Delayed stress is more difficult to recognize than acute stress. So much time may have passed that the person experiencing the delayed stress may not associate it with the original critical incident. In addition, the passage of time has a way of distorting, adding to, covering, or exaggerating the typical symptoms, and this contributes to the difficulties usually associated with recognizing stress reactions.[19]

Delayed stress is more tenacious than acute stress. That is, it is much harder to resolve. It has been around a longer time and thus has had more time to establish roots. In many cases psychological support from a professional therapist may be necessary to break the problems encountered by a person caught up in the web of delayed stress. (Recognition signs and symptoms are presented in Chapter 3, and preventive or recovery strategies and techniques are given in Chapters 4, 5, and 6.)

POST TRAUMATIC STRESS DISORDER

It has already been stated in a number of ways that people's reactions to stressful events are normal. That theme will be repeated numerous times throughout this book since both authors are firm believers in the concept that normal people have normal (although painful) reactions to abnormal events.

However, when emergency workers resort to excessive suppression of their emotions and when they avoid preventive strategies such as psychological debriefings (see Chapter 5) after a traumatic event they may be setting themselves up for a potentially serious condition called Post Traumatic Stress Disorder (PTSD). Post Traumatic Stress Disorder is beyond the "normal" response to stress. It occurs when people cannot (or, in some cases, will not) work through their normal reactions and recover from the awful experience. They get stuck and life for them is changed. They suffer emotionally and sometimes physically as a result of powerful stressors that have invaded their lives. The condition is frequently permanent.

Post Traumatic Stress Disorder is not something to be taken lightly. It is a serious condition that can lead to personality changes, illness, and if it is ignored, may end with the person's suicide. PTSD is the abnormal end result of a powerful and overwhelming stressful incident. It is considered a pathological state, *not* a normal state. Something has gone very wrong and the person is not able to recover from the traumatic event. PTSD is a diagnosis that can be made only by psychiatrists, psychologists, and other mental health professionals. It is not a matter for self-diagnosis; it requires professional evaluations. PTSD is an anxiety disorder. Anxiety disorders are one of the three main groups of mental disorders. PTSD is called a disorder because it disrupts the normal functions of one's life. The disorder interferes with sleep, activities, relationships with others, and even with one's health.

However, PTSD is not a psychosis (the group of the most serious forms of mental disturbance). Instead, it is listed as an "anxiety" disorder because some of its chief characteristics are anxiety, fear, apprehension, and avoidance of painful stimuli.[20]

Unfortunately, about 4 percent (a rough estimate) of emergency personnel who are exposed to a powerfully distressing incident may develop the disorder, which is characterized by a vivid reexperiencing of the terrible event, numbed emotions, startle responses, and avoidance of activities or other stimuli that remind a person of the awful circumstances they experienced. That 4 percent figure could easily be reduced substantially if organizations and individuals would simply follow some of the preventive stress management strategies recommended in Chapters 4, 5, and 6.[21,22]

A diagnosis of Post Traumatic Stress Disorder should be made only by trained mental health professionals who are very familiar with the disorder. The amateur is likely to misdiagnose the problem. Emergency workers faced with the wrong type of mental health services would almost be better off with no mental health services at all. This is especially so when PTSD is involved. The proper treatment of the condition requires a knowledgeable and skilled mental health professional.

Here are some guidelines from the American Psychiatric Association's publication, *Diagnostic and Statistical Manual of Mental Disorders,* 3rd edition, revised, 1987. These guidelines are presented here only to assist emergency personnel if a formal diagnosis of PTSD and professional treatment appears to be indicated for themselves or for another.

To have PTSD, an emergency responder must have been exposed to a highly traumatic event that would be unusual and extremely distressing to almost anyone exposed to it, such as seeing someone killed as a result of a violent act or serious accident, or a significant threat to one's own life or to the lives of a spouse or one's children. Destruction of a person's home or community are also conditions that may set the stage for the eventual development of PTSD. The event must be excessively demanding, overwhelming, disgusting, or terrifying, or it will not be powerful enough to produce PTSD.

The diagnosis of PTSD can be made only if the signs and symptoms of disturbance from a particularly bad event last a month or more. Symptoms that are commonly found in PTSD may exist in emergency workers shortly after the event, but true PTSD is not given as a diagnosis unless the disorder lasts beyond a month.

PTSD is best recognized by its primary characteristics. They are:

1. A disturbing event that is well outside the range of usual human experience.

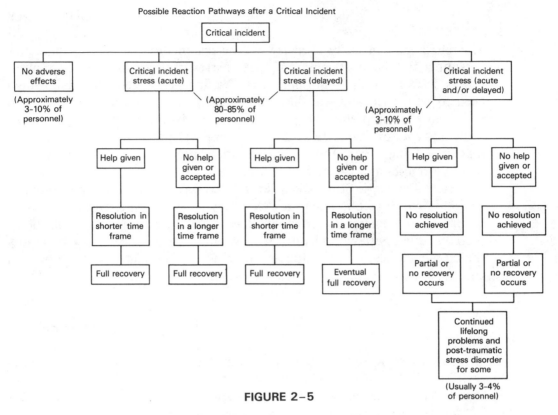

FIGURE 2-5

2. The person reexperiences the event in his or her thoughts, dreams, or daily life (flashbacks).
3. The person avoids any stimuli associated with the event and numbs his or her emotions.
4. Physical, emotional, cognitive, and behavioral signs and symptoms which were not present prior to the event and which have lasted longer than a month.

If the signs and symptoms of distress do not show up for six months or more after the stressful event, the diagnosis becomes *Post Traumatic Stress Disorder—delayed.*

If you recognize yourself or another person in a majority of the signs of PTSD described above, further evaluation and possibly psychological treatment may be indicated. It is strongly recommended that you not take risks with your health and happiness. Instead, search out appropriate mental health personnel who can help you to work through the PTSD and thus return to a more normal, fulfilling, and happy life experience.[23] (Additional information on PTSD is presented in Chapter 3.) Figure 2-5 describes various pathways that stress reactions may follow.

SUMMARY

This chapter involves an overview of the personality profile of emergency personnel and the most common types of stress they are likely to encounter. It was shown that action-oriented, risk-taking personnel who have a high need to be needed and who like immediate gratification are very likely to put themselves into emergency work and thus be more frequently exposed to acute types of stress. In addition, emergency personnel have a difficult time expressing their emotions and are more prone to experiencing delayed stress responses and the effects of cumulative stress.

Post Traumatic Stress Disorder (PTSD) was described as a pathological end state which results from an excessively stressful experience. That is, it occurs when a person is so overwhelmed by a powerful incident that he or she is unable to recover adequately. PTSD can be managed only by highly skilled mental health professionals who are very familiar with the condition and the special treatment needs of those who develop it.

REFERENCES

1. Graham, N. K. (1981). Done in, fed up, burned out: Too much attrition in EMS. *Journal of Emergency Medical Services, 6*(1): 24.
2. Maslach, C., and Jackson, S. (1979). Burned out cops and their families. *Psychology Today,* May, 59.
3. Robinson, R. (1986). *Health and Stress in Ambulance Services.* Melbourne, Australia: Social Biology Resources Centre.
4. Hurrell, J. J., Pate, A., and Kheisnnet, R. (1984). *Stress among Police Officers,* Pub. 84-108. Washington, DC: National Institute for Occupational Safety and Health, U.S. Department of Health and Human Services.
5. Mitchell, J. T. (1986). Living dangerously: Why fire fighters take risks. *Firehouse, 11*(8): 50–51; 63.
6. Graham, N. K. (1981). How to avoid a short career. *Journal of Emergency Medical Services, 6*(2): 25.
7. Everly, G. S., and Mitchell, J. T. Unpublished study.
8. Schonpflug, W. (1986). Behavior economics as an approach to stress theory. In M. H. Appley and R. Trumbull (Eds.), *Dynamics of Stress: Physiological, Psychological and Social Perspectives.* New York: Plenum, pp. 81–98.
9. Munn, H. E., and Metzger, N. (1981). *Effective Communication in Health Care: A Supervisor's Handbook.* Rockville, MD: Aspen Systems Corporation.
10. Friedman, M., and Roseman, R. (1974). *Type A Behavior and Your Heart.* New York: Alfred A. Knopf.

11. Farber, B. A. (1983). A critical perspective on burnout. *Stress and Burnout in the Human Service Profession.* New York: Pergamon Press, pp. 1–20.

12. Freudenberger, H. J. (1974). Staff burnout. *Journal of Social Issues, 30,* 159–165.

13. Patrick, P. K. (1981). *Health Care Worker Burnout: What It Is, What to Do about It.* Chicago: Inquiry Books.

14. Maslach, C. (1976). Burned out. *Human Behavior, 5,* 16–22.

15. Pines, A., and Aronson, E., with Kafry, D. (1981). *Burnout: From Tedium to Personal Growth.* New York: Free Press.

16. Flannery, R. (1987). From victim to survivor: A stress management approach in the treatment of learned helplessness. In B. A. van der Kolk (Ed.), *Psychological Trauma.* Washington, DC: American Psychiatric Press, pp. 217–232.

17. Mitchell, J. T. (1985). Healing the helper. In B. Green (Ed.), *Role Stressors and Supports for Emergency Workers.* Washington, DC: Center for Mental Health Studies of Emergencies, U.S. Department of Health and Human Services.

18. Mitchell, J. T. (1983). When disaster strikes: The critical incident stress debriefing process. *Journal of Emergency Medical Services, 8*(1): 36–39.

19. Mitchell, J. T. (1986). *Critical incident stress management. Response,* Sept./ Oct., 24–25.

20. American Psychiatric Association. (1987). Post-traumatic stress disorder. *Diagnostic and Statistical Manual of Mental Disorders,* 3rd ed., rev. (DSM-III-R). Washington, DC: APA.

21. Scrignar, C. B. (1984). *Post Traumatic Stress Disorder: Diagnosis, Treatment, and Legal Issues.* New York: Praeger.

22. Scrignar, C. B. (1983). *Stress Strategies: The Treatment of the Anxiety Disorders.* Basel: Karger.

23. Everly, G. S. (1989). *A Clinical Guide to the Treatment of Human Stress.* New York: Plenum.

3

DISTRESS SIGNALS

Acute, delayed, or cumulative stress reactions all display signals by which they can be recognized. The distress signals are, at times, easy to notice even when observed only casually. Seeing a person punch a wall would be a good example. But sometimes, distress signals are more subtle and remain camouflaged behind a variety of distracting behaviors, communications, and issues. A minor increase in silence on the part of an emergency worker is a subtle sign that may have many meanings. Such a change may not be so obvious to those who work with the person.

Signals of distress are always present and can be found when someone knows what to look for and where to look. Missed distress signals in oneself or a fellow worker may have disastrous consequences. In this chapter we cover the basic distress signals that emergency personnel should recognize if they wish to prevent stress-related problems in their own lives and those of their fellow workers.

SIGNALS OF DISTRESS

Distress signals are indications that corrective action is needed. They are often called signs or symptoms. Unfortunately, those words have usually been applied to sick people or to their illnesses. Since emergency people do not like to be considered sick, they balk at the words and are uncomfortable when the words are applied to them or to their signals of distress. However, the words ''signs'' and ''symptoms'' are applied to healthy people as well. A *sign* is something that indicates the presence of something else. The sign is usually obvious to an observer. When you see an emergency worker who usually performs very well now wandering around aimlessly, you are seeing a sign of distress.

A *symptom* also indicates the presence of something else. However, it is more subtle than a sign and usually needs to be reported by the person who is experiencing it. If someone were to tell you that he was feeling confused, he would be reporting a symptom. In the examples just presented, neither the sign nor the symptom indicates illness or craziness. In fact, most signs and symptoms of stress are normal reactions to unusual circumstances. They indicate merely a state of distress—not weakness, mental disturbance, nor incompetence. They are signals that corrective action may be necessary if further consequences are going to be prevented.[1]

Degrees of Intensity

Highway warning signs, alarm bells, and whistles come in various shapes and sizes, have brighter or more subdued colors, and flash, ring, or sound at various levels depending on the urgency of the warning. Similarly, signals of human distress may have various levels of intensity, depending on the severity of the stress reaction. A very mild stressful event produces a mild stress reaction and set of distress signals which may be barely noticeable. As the intensity of the stressful situation increases, so does the intensity of the stress signals that are experienced or displayed. The greater the number and intensity of the distress signals, the more need there is for emergency personnel to recognize them quickly and respond actively and effectively. Moderate-to-severe stress signs and symptoms, when ignored or denied excessively, are almost certain to generate illness or other forms of disruption in most human beings. Emergency personnel are no exception.[2]

Change

All too often, emergency personnel tend to deny or ignore one of the most significant distress signals—*change*. Ignoring or denying changes in themselves or in others is a dangerous activity since the type and degree of change indicate the level of disruption produced by acute, delayed, and cumulative stress reactions. Change in an individual or a group may be noticed in four major areas. Changes may occur in an emergency person's (1) *body or general health,* and changes may also occur in the way in which a person (2) *thinks,* (3) *feels,* and/or (4) *acts.* Any significant change in one of the four major areas or a series of changes in one or more of the areas should be taken seriously as a distress signal. The greater the number of changes noticed in an emergency person, the greater the level of distress.

Changes that signal distress may be temporary, which is usually the case for emergency personnel who are experiencing an acute or delayed reaction. Understanding and support from officers and other concerned people and personal actions designed to lessen stress reactions (see Chapters 4, 5, and 6) improve the chances of rapid recovery and usually help emergency personnel to eliminate the signals of distress and restore themselves to their normal health, feelings, thoughts, and usual activities.[3]

At times, changes become permanent. This is particularly common in the cumulative or chronic stress reactions described in Chapter 2. It takes a great deal of energy to turn a permanent change around. Most people will need help from a physician if the change is a physical one or from a mental health professional if the change has occurred in the emergency person's thinking process, emotions, or behaviors (see Chapters 4 and 5). Quick action in response to a significant change in an individual or a group may prevent changes from becoming permanent. Response to the early warning signals of distress may actually mitigate or eliminate the cumulative stress response and the difficulties associated with recovering from that type of chronic stress.

Emergency personnel are therefore urged to notice and react to stress-related changes in themselves or the people in their units. Denial of the changes or a false belief that the changes will simply disappear by themselves is a dangerous game to play.

WARNING SIGNALS OF ACUTE STRESS

During critical incidents there are many warning signals of acute stress reactions, as noted in Tables 3–1 and 3–2. It is not necessary for a person to have all or even a number of the signs and symptoms listed to be considered in the midst of a stress reaction. A handful of signs and symptoms from one or more of the four main categories in each table would be sufficient to assess the degree of intensity of the warning signals. Then appropriate responses to the warnings may be developed based on the needs of the person or group involved in the stressful event. Considerable information that is useful in reducing emergency service stress is presented in Chapters 4, 5, and 6.

These signs and symptoms are primarily warning signals; they do not necessarily indicate physical or mental illness. Signals of stress do not indicate weakness. They are normal in every way; they simply indicate a need for corrective action to limit the impact of a stressful event or to begin the recovery process.[4,5]

The signs and symptoms in the tables usually appear during the emergency response or within a 24-hour period. Under special circumstances, they may be delayed for hours, days, weeks, months, and years. The warning signals listed in Table 3-1 are the most significant and require immediate corrective action.[6-9] Those in Table 3-2 are common but usually demand less immediate attention.[11-15]

Remember, the existence of many of the signs and symptoms in Table 3-1 is a serious distress signal and demands immediate attention. There may be many other signs and symptoms which indicate the presence of a significant stress reaction. Table 3-2 provides a list of the most common of these.

Some signs or symptoms from each of the four areas listed (physical, cognitive, emotional, behavioral) are usually present in either an acute or a delayed stress reaction. There may be other stress symptoms that do not appear in the tables. Stress has been known to produce an enormous variety

TABLE 3-1 Distress Signals Requiring Immediate Corrective Action

PHYSICAL	COGNITIVE
Chest pain*	Decreased alertness to surroundings
Difficulty breathing*	Difficulties making decisions
Excessive blood pressure*	Hyper alertness
Collapse from exhaustion*	Generalized mental confusion
Cardiac arrythmias*	Disorientation to person, place, time
Signs of severe shock*	Serious disruption in thinking
Excessive dehydration*	Seriously slowed thinking
Dizziness*	Problems in naming familiar items
Excessive vomiting*	Problem recognizing familiar people
Blood in stool*	

EMOTIONAL	BEHAVIORAL
Panic reactions	Significant change in speech patterns
Shock-like state	Excessively angry outbursts
Phobic reaction	Crying spells
General loss of control	Antisocial acts (e.g., violence)
Inappropriate emotions	Extreme hyperactivity

*Indicates a need for medical evaluation.

TABLE 3–2   Common Signs and Symptoms
of Distress Not Requiring Immediate Action

PHYSICAL	COGNITIVE
Nausea	Confusion
Upset stomach	Lowered attention span
Tremors (lips, hands)	Calculation difficulties
Feeling uncoordinated	Memory problems
Profuse sweating	Poor concentration
Chills	Seeing an event over and over
Diarrhea	Distressing dreams
Rapid heart rate	Disruption in logical thinking
Muscle aches	Blaming someone
Sleep disturbance	
Dry mouth	
Shakes	
Vision problems	
Fatigue	

EMOTIONAL	BEHAVIORAL
Anticipatory anxiety	Change in activity
Denial	Withdrawal
Fear	Suspiciousness
Survivor guilt	Change in communications
Uncertainty of feelings	Change in interactions with others
Depression	Increased or decreased food intake
Grief	Increased smoking
Feeling hopeless	Increased alcohol intake
Feeling overwhelmed	Overly vigilant to environment
Feeling lost	Excessive humor
Feeling abandoned	Excessive silence
Worried	Unusual behavior
Wishing to hide	
Wishing to die	
Anger	
Feeling numb	
Identifying with victim	

of signs and symptoms. A complete list of stress signs and symptoms would be burdensome to read and would not serve a useful purpose.[10] If you wish to learn more about stress signs and symptoms, it is recommended that you consult the books and articles listed at the end of the chapter.

In addition to those marked in Table 3–1 as requiring medical attention, any signs or symptoms that become severe or are not relieved by rest or support from others should be evaluated further by appropriate medical or psychological professionals.

As stated earlier, these signs and symptoms do not usually indicate mental illness. But any preexisting problem(s), including mental illness, may be made worse by a stressful event.

SIGNS OF DELAYED STRESS

A great many people have little or no noticeable reaction to stress at the scene. Their reactions tend to show up days or weeks after the event has passed, but the signs and symptoms of stress are just as real and painful as they would be if they occurred at the time of or shortly after the crisis event. However, because of the time lapse, the signs and symptoms are more confusing. They feel out of place to people who have returned to their everyday tasks and thought they had put a bad incident behind them. Some emergency personnel are unable to identify any connection between a past bad event and their current signs and symptoms. That inability to see a connection between past events and current reactions often makes them increasingly vulnerable to more significant risks to their health and happiness.

Intrusive Images

Delayed stress reactions are often recognized by the existence of intrusive images. Intrusive images may appear in the form of bothersome thoughts which have a tendency to come into a person's mind when they are least welcome. They can get in the way and cause a person to experience difficulties with attention span, concentration, and other mental functions. They are generally distracting thoughts that relate to the distressing incident. When intrusive thoughts are present, a person may feel the same anxiety and discomfort which was present at the scene during the event.[16]

Intrusive images may also show up as daydreams or nightmares. The visual and auditory images are usually quite vivid representations of the critical incident. They may be dreams that replay the incident exactly as it occurred in real life or they may be bizarre distortions of reality. Frequently, dreams about a bad situation or an awful scene are so powerful that they can wake someone from a sound sleep. Dreams can be so distressing that they produce physiological responses such as sweating, muscle twitches, or an upset stomach.

Another way that intrusive images tend to show up is through auditory, visual, or olfactory (smell, taste) impulses. People who have been through a bad scene may reexperience smells such as the smell of death, blood, feces, gun powder, jet fuel, or other noxious odors even when they are nowhere near anything that would stimulate such odors. They may also see some aspects of the situation over and over in their mind's eye. Some people hear sounds that occurred during the incident.

Sights, smells, and sounds associated with an emergency incident which occur later when people are away from the scene and awake are called *flashbacks*. Flashbacks are like a dream except that the person is fully awake. They are a sign that the person's mind is trying to work through the event in an effort to make sense of it.

There is mounting evidence that traumatic events may be powerful enough to imprint themselves in the biochemistry of the brain. A slight stimulus may trigger a biochemical reaction in the brain, which in turn initiates all the thoughts and emotions and sometimes even the physical responses that were present during the actual incident. Researchers believe that the process may be somewhat similar to the imprinting process that takes place in the presence of hallucinogenic drugs such as PCP or LSD. Even though the drug is not currently present in a person's system, he or she may have auditory, visual, and olfactory flashbacks as well as emotional reactions. Similarly, even though the situation is long past, flashbacks continue to occur without any form of provocation because the chemistry of the brain may have been affected during the stressful event.[17,18]

Intrusive images such as obsessive thoughts about an incident, flashbacks, daydreams, and nightmares are often distressing, but they are *not* usually signs of weakness or psychosis in emergency personnel. They are a normal part of the process of working through an awful situation. Talking about intrusive images to a mental health professional or a well-trained peer support person who is familiar with traumatic stress responses usually makes them subside more rapidly and helps to put them in perspective.

Physical Signs

Intrusive images are not the only signs of delayed stress. There are many physical signs as well. Sleep disturbance is probably the most common. Emergency people who have experienced a stressful event often have trouble sleeping. Some have trouble falling asleep, while others wake up a number of times during the night or have disturbing dreams that interfere with sleep. Other people wake up early or wake up in the morning feeling fatigued.

Some emergency workers break out in a cold sweat even months after a critical incident when something reminds them of the event. They may also experience nausea, muscle tremors, and startle responses. Loud noises, odors, and certain sights may cause dramatic reactions in emergency personnel who are suffering from delayed stress reactions.[19]

Occasionally, emergency workers experience lowered sexual drive or an inability to perform sexually as a result of delayed stress reactions. They may also become more resistant to touching or being touched after a delayed stress reaction begins. This, of course has very negative effects on spouses, children, and friends, who wonder what has gone wrong.

It is not uncommon for emergency personnel to develop diseases after experiencing a traumatic event. Ulcers, coronary artery disease, diabetes, and cancer have been known to appear in people who have experienced terrible things in the course of their work.

It takes a thorough medical and psychological evaluation to establish a link between traumatic events and the development of disease. If an emergency services person believes that he or she has a stress-related disease, it is advised that the person avoid self-diagnosis and arrange for a complete evaluation by professionals.

Emotional Signs

The emotional response to delayed stress is often covert (hidden). The person cannot recognize what is actually creating the strong emotional reactions. Frequently, emergency personnel say such things as: "I don't understand why I am feeling like this. I've had worse calls before and they never bothered me as much as this one." Such a response is often a reaction to one or more of their earlier "worse" calls. The current call may be simply the trigger mechanism that stirred up the feelings associated with the earlier call(s). The combined emotions of both the earlier call(s) and the current one become so overpowering that the usual ability of an emergency worker to deal effectively with a single incident is seriously disrupted. At times the help of a counselor may be quite useful in sorting out all the feelings from all the calls and in resolving the true source of the person's current reactions.

Long after an event has passed, emergency personnel may experience intense feelings of depression or a loss of emotional control. They are usually pretty surprised when intense emotions hit them weeks, months, or a year or more after an incident. They do not see any connection between what happened in the past and how they are feeling now, but the connection is there.

Feelings of intense grief and depression are the most common emotional signals of delayed stress reactions. Virtually without warning an emergency worker may feel overcome by deep grief or depression. They could be typing a report that is unrelated to the distressing incident or simply watching television or reading a newspaper. They may suddenly cry or feel torn apart inside for reasons that are not obvious to them. They do not realize that as an emergency worker, they responded very well to some event in the past, but as a person, as a human being, they were wounded and never realized it.[20]

One of the most common emotional signs of a delayed stress reaction is a growing sense of isolation. There may be a feeling that "no one understands what I'm going through" or a fear that the person will always be alone or "different" from everybody else. Emergency personnel usually feel a sense of belonging within the emergency services in which they work. There is something of a brotherhood in the services—almost an extended family. When people feel isolated from the "family," they experience a considerable amount of pain, fear, and anxiety.

Frequently, we develop such feelings of aloneness because of guilt or self-doubt following a difficult call. Emergency responders are experts at dissecting every action or decision and putting themselves down for any possible mistake. Picking at actions, decisions, and mistakes produces heightened feelings of guilt, self-doubt, and obsessions with mistakes.

Anger, irritability, and rage are very common manifestations of delayed stress. Anger and rage and the irritability that accompany them are defensive reactions designed to keep other people at a distance and to limit the demands of the environment on the distressed person. Anger is usually a secondary emotion closely linked to frustration and disappointment. Anger may also be turned inward against oneself if a person believes that he or she has a significant degree of responsibility for something that went wrong.[21]

Other emotions that come to the surface long after a traumatic event are a sense of hopelessness and purposelessness or despair. Many emergency workers lose a sense of the future and are unable to make sense out of their current world. They may feel lost and abandoned.

General anxiety and fear of future events may also develop in traumatized emergency workers. They become concerned that when similar events occur, they may not be able to manage themselves adequately.

If a specific event went bad and the emergency worker made a mistake during the incident, he or she may feel so guilty that they are unable to continue in emergency services. Frequently, guilt feelings eat away at the self-esteem of such persons. They become defensive about their ability and react strongly to minor stimuli.

Feelings of guilt, despair, anxiety, hopelessness, and anger at oneself which are out of control may eventually produce suicidal thinking. Hopefully, a distressed emergency worker will seek professional help (or be ordered to do so if that becomes necessary) before he or she is able to act on such feelings.[22]

Cognitive Signs

Sometimes delayed stress manifests itself as a deterioration in an emergency worker's thinking processes. Mental confusion may develop, along with a lowered attention span. It may become more difficult for the person to make decisions or to perform problem-solving activities.

Many emergency personnel experience intense distractibility in their work weeks after a critical incident. It is as if they have lost the ability to filter out unnecessary stimuli. They lose their ability to concentrate. They can no longer sort things out as they had in the past.[23]

At times some emergency workers begin repetitive obsessive thinking patterns which they find difficult to break. These thoughts are often about specific elements of the traumatic incident. Some report that their thinking becomes narrowed so that they are unable to pay attention to other aspects of their life. They develop tunnel vision—the only thing they are able to think about is the critical incident.

Constant internal reminders of a critical incident stir up some of the emotions and physical reactions that were described earlier. The emotions stirred by the constant reminders may contribute to changes in a person's behavior.

Behavioral Signs

Delayed stress reactions also show up in a person's behavior. Behaviors are the side effects of a mixture of physical, emotional, and cognitive factors. For example, if an emergency person thinks that he or she made a serious mistake during an incident, guilt feelings may evolve which cause the person to experience nausea, muscle tremors, and a startle reflex. The cognitive, emotional, and physical reactions combine and show up in the person's behavior. That is, he or she may avoid contact with superior officers in the unit or may not show up for a variety of unit functions.

Unfortunately, distressed emergency workers also tend to avoid contact with the people who love them most and who might provide the best support. They tend to cut off contact with their spouses, children, and extended family members. Parents and brothers and sisters also get caught in the cut-off process. Not only are they not in contact with relatives and friends; they also refuse to discuss anything with them. Those who would support them are left feeling helpless and severely limited in what they might be able to do to help. Frequently, as communications fail, the loved ones begin to blame themselves for whatever has gone wrong between them and the loved one. The family members begin to be penalized because the response person is suffering.

This unfair penalizing of family members can be eliminated if the emergency person will step back for a moment and see what is happening to them. Admitting that one may be experiencing a delayed stress reaction often gets a person on a new track in which they can seek out trusted people in their lives and open up the communications. Good friends, family members, members of the clergy, and counselors may be very helpful in restoring balance to the worker's life.

Withdrawal from contact with others is one of the most common behavioral manifestations of delayed stress. But there are also other behavioral signals of delayed stress reactions.[24] Angry outbursts toward family members, friends, and fellow workers is one of the behavioral signs of delayed stress. So is the development of suspiciousness in one's dealings with others. Some people with delayed stress will become very silent. Others become extremely talkative or make excessive attempts to be funny.

The important point to note is that current behavior is changed substantially from previous behavior. The behavior that is now being demonstrated by fellow workers is unusual and in some way less effective or efficient. It is especially important to note any destructive behavior, such as increased use of alcohol or tobacco. Rapid, unnecessary, or extreme decisions that are not in the person's best interest may be highly significant signals of delayed stress. People should be urged to slow down their rapid-fire decisions and their reactions so that they do not make rash decisions or take actions that may eventually work against them.

If a person is having a great deal of difficulty sorting out delayed stress, they should seek help from someone they love or from a professional.

RECOGNIZING POST TRAUMATIC STRESS DISORDER

To reiterate some concepts already presented in Chapter 2, experiencing a critical incident does not necessarily mean that a person is going to develop Post Traumatic Stress Disorder (PTSD). Most emergency personnel (in fact, better than 86 percent) who go through a critical incident will experience acute and/or delayed stress reactions[25]; that is, they have cognitive, emotional, physical, or behavioral side effects to the incident. However, either by themselves or with some help from friends or professionals, most emergency personnel are able to recover fully from a critical incident. Their signs and symptoms gradually subside with the passage of time, or they work them out.

But when a critical incident is extremely powerful, when it is well outside the usual range of human experience, it may cause PTSD to develop in a small number of people who experienced the event. There is no way to predict who is going to be affected sufficiently by a powerful event to produce PTSD. The occurrence of PTSD seems to be somewhat random. Some people develop PTSD, others manage to escape it; roughly 4 percent of emergency personnel suffer from PTSD. Many factors are present that contribute to its development:[17,18,26]

1. How closely is an individual involved with the event? The majority of torture victims, for example, develop PTSD. A much smaller number of those who only witnessed the torture will develop PTSD.
2. What experience has the person had in dealing with excessively stressful events?
3. What is going on in the person's current life? Illness in a loved one, pregnancy, a recent death of a loved one, or some other traumatic event may set the stage for the development of PTSD.
4. What hidden meaning does a particular incident have for the emergency worker? Does it produce powerful frightening memories from childhood?
5. What past unresolved losses or traumas are stored up inside one's mind?
6. How anxious is the person in general?
7. How much help was available immediately after the event, and how receptive was the person to that help?
8. How fast was help available?
9. How supportive were fellow workers and superiors?
10. How helpful and supportive was the person's family after the incident? How open was communications with loved ones?

Post Traumatic Stress Disorder has many characteristic signs and symptoms. People who suffer from it often have many of the following conditions:[27]

-   Disturbing memories of the event which pop to mind unexpectedly
-   Dreams or nightmares related to the incident
-   Feeling as if the event were happening again

- Psychological distress around the anniversary of the trauma
- Numbing of one's emotions
- Avoidance of thoughts or feelings associated with the event
- Avoidance of activities that recall the incident
- Loss of memory associated with important aspects of the event
- Loss of interest in activities previously enjoyed
- Feeling detached and estranged from others
- Loss of loving feelings toward others
- A sense of a shortened future
- Difficulty falling asleep and staying asleep
- Intense irritability
- Difficulty concentrating
- Startle reflexes
- Excessive suspicion and caution in dealing with others
- Physical reactions in circumstances similar to the original incident
- Feeling keyed up and unable to relax
- Loss of emotional control

If you have experienced a single, extraordinary past event or a series of events that you found very distressing, and if you notice that you have a number of the signs and symptoms presented above which started during or after the incident, you may be suffering from Post Traumatic Stress Disorder. If the emergency event(s) haunts you and is interfering with your life or with important aspects of your life, you would be well advised to seek out at least an evaluation by a mental health professional. PTSD does not just disappear by itself. It may hang on indefinitely and produce unbelievable disruption in your life. Alcoholism, marital or relationship discord, personality changes, loss of one's career, and even suicide may result if you ignore PTSD. In short, the very best advice that can be given to anyone who is suffering the after effects of a terrible event and suspects that it might be PTSD is to *get help*.

SIGNS OF CUMULATIVE STRESS

Cumulative stress occurs as a result of prolonged exposure to a great many stressors over a long period of time. The stressors do not necessarily have to be severe, as is the case with an acute or critical incident stress. *Cumu-*

lative stress is usually caused by a combination of a wide range of work and nonwork stressors.[28]

Recognition of a cumulative stress reaction is not easy. The condition is slow to develop (usually taking several years to manifest itself). It is an extremely complex form of stress, with many subtle signs that are easy to confuse with a number of other conditions. By the time it is noticed, permanent damage to a person's health and happiness may have been sustained.

Descriptions of the signs and symptoms of the cumulative stress phases presented in the following sections may be helpful to emergency personnel who wish to recognize a cumulative stress reaction in themselves or others while there is still time to make a positive change. Cumulative stress reactions can be experienced in four relatively distinct phases:[28]

1. Warning phase
2. Mild symptom phase
3. Entrenched phase
4. Severe/debilitating phase

Phase 1: Warning

The warning signs of an impending cumulative stress reaction are predominantly emotional in nature. They may take a year or more to grow to any noticeable degree. The earliest signs of a cumulative stress reaction are feelings of:

- Vague anxiety
- Depression
- Boredom
- Apathy
- Emotional fatigue

Noticing the early warning signs of cumulative stress and taking immediate action to reverse them assures a rapid recovery and a blockage of further development of the cumulative stress reaction. Frequently, all that is necessary is a change of activity, a vacation, or open discussions with supervisors, family members, and friends. Taking more time for oneself and combining relaxation and rest time may go far to reverse the early warning signs of a cumulative stress reaction. In emergency work, changing one's assignment may be one of the most helpful early strategies.

Phase 2: Mild Symptoms

If neglected or ignored, the warning signals of cumulative stress become fixed and intensify. Over a time frame of about six to eighteen months a person who is moving deeper into a cumulative stress reaction begins to show additional signs of distress. All of the symptoms of the warning phase continue. However, some physical signs become coupled with the emotional signs described in phase 1. Some of the more common signs and symptoms in the second phase are:

- More frequent loss of emotional control
- Sleep disturbances
- More frequent headaches, colds, and/or stomach problems
- Muscle aches
- Intensified physical and emotional fatigue
- Withdrawal from contact with others
- Irritability
- Intensifying depression

It is still possible to reduce or eliminate the growing cumulative stress reaction, but the person must be much more aggressive in making a life-style change. Such people need more balance in their work and home life. Reduction of stress in every area of life is a necessity. Many emergency personnel would benefit from some short-term counseling (for one to three months) when they are struggling with the intensifying symptoms of cumulative stress response. See Chapters 4, 5, and 6 for more details on strategies to cut back on stress so that life becomes more balanced.

Phase 3: Entrenched Cumulative Stress Reaction

To reach phase 3 of the cumulative stress reaction, people have to have ignored blatantly the previous two phases in which many subtle and some obvious signs and symptoms of distress evolved. Once a cumulative stress reaction becomes entrenched or fixed solidly in place, it is very difficult to make changes that would balance the person's physical and emotional systems. People who have allowed a cumulative stress reaction to become entrenched will be suffering through some of the most painful conditions they have ever encountered in their life. Their careers, family life, and personal happiness are on the line and immediate efforts to get help and lower their stress are essential. They will normally experience at least some of the following signs and symptoms:[29-31]

- Skin rashes
- General physical and emotional fatigue
- Intense depression
- Increased alcohol use
- Use of nonprescription drugs
- Increased smoking
- Elevated blood pressure
- Migraine headaches
- Poor appetite
- Loss of sexual drive
- Ulcers
- Intense irritability
- Marital discord or relationship problems
- Crying spells
- Intense anxiety
- Cardiac problems
- Rigid thinking
- Withdrawal from friends, family, and coworkers
- Restlessness
- Sleeplessness
- Other physical and emotional symptoms

In most cases people do not get out of a phase 3 cumulative stress reaction without some help from medical and psychological professionals.

If life is getting tougher to handle with each passing day, *get help now.*

Phase 4: Severe/Debilitating Cumulative Stress Reaction

Allowing oneself to deteriorate so much that one enters phase 4 of the cumulative stress reactions is a clear indication that a person cannot or will not pay attention to a great many signals of distress in his or her lives. At times the presence of a phase 4 cumulative stress reaction may suggest that the person is, in fact, self-destructive. Professional help is a necessity if that is the case.

Usually after five to ten years of ignoring signs and symptoms of growing stress problems and refusing to do anything to correct the cumulative stress reaction, people enter the ultimately destructive final phase. If they somehow manage to survive this phase, they are rarely able to continue working in the same field. Their careers end prematurely. So do their lives. They are usually quite sick, both emotionally and physically. They almost always need significant intervention from professionals. The signs and symptoms that began in phases 1 through 3 continue into phase 4 and become intensified.

Most people who have neglected themselves enough to end up in a phase 4 cumulative stress reaction will have a number of the following *severe signs and symptoms of cumulative stress:*[29–33]

- Asthma
- Coronary artery disease
- Heart attacks
- Diabetes
- Cancer
- Severe emotional depression
- Lowered self-esteem
- Lowered self-confidence
- Inability to perform one's job
- Inability to manage one's personal life
- Severe withdrawal
- Uncontrolled emotions: anger, grief, rage
- Suicidal or homicidal thinking
- Muscle tremors
- Extreme chronic fatigue
- Over reactions to minor events
- Agitation
- Chronic feelings of tension
- Poor concentration and attention span
- Frequent accidents
- Carelessness
- Forgetfulness
- Feelings of hostility
- Intense feelings of paranoia
- Moderate to severe thought disorders
- Other severe physical and emotional signs and symptoms

The cumulative stress reaction usually takes from one to ten years to develop fully. It is almost totally preventable if people take sufficient care of themselves, know the danger signs, and are ready to keep their work and home lives in a state of balance.

Prevention of cumulative stress should be the major emphasis in cumulative stress reactions. It is obviously a far better thing to do to prevent the development of the problems associated with a cumulative stress than to try to cure the condition once it develops. Many of the suggestions in the chapters to follow will be of great use to emergency personnel who wish to reduce their chances of cumulative stress and all its complications. Take action now to cut down the potential for big losses later.

CUMULATIVE STRESS TEST

Dr. Herbert J. Freudenberger has developed a simple test which can help to determine if a person is developing cumulative stress reactions (see Figure 3-1). He suggests that a person review the changes in his or her life during the past few months. Think about each question for a brief period (30 sec-

---

FIGURE 3-1 Firewatch

1 = no change
2 = little change
3 = moderate change
4 = considerable change
5 = a great deal of change

_____ 1. Do you tire more easily? Feel fatigued rather than energetic?

_____ 2. Are people annoying you by telling you, "You don't look so good lately"?

_____ 3. Are you working harder and harder and accomplishing less and less?

_____ 4. Are you increasingly cynical and disenchanted?

_____ 5. Are you often invaded by a sadness you cannot explain?

_____ 6. Are you forgetting appointments, deadlines, personal possessions?

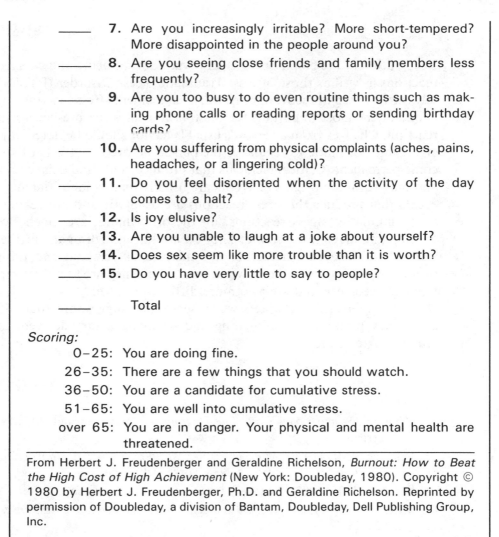

_____ 7. Are you increasingly irritable? More short-tempered? More disappointed in the people around you?

_____ 8. Are you seeing close friends and family members less frequently?

_____ 9. Are you too busy to do even routine things such as making phone calls or reading reports or sending birthday cards?

_____ 10. Are you suffering from physical complaints (aches, pains, headaches, or a lingering cold)?

_____ 11. Do you feel disoriented when the activity of the day comes to a halt?

_____ 12. Is joy elusive?

_____ 13. Are you unable to laugh at a joke about yourself?

_____ 14. Does sex seem like more trouble than it is worth?

_____ 15. Do you have very little to say to people?

_____   Total

Scoring:
    0–25: You are doing fine.
   26–35: There are a few things that you should watch.
   36–50: You are a candidate for cumulative stress.
   51–65: You are well into cumulative stress.
   over 65: You are in danger. Your physical and mental health are threatened.

From Herbert J. Freudenberger and Geraldine Richelson, _Burnout: How to Beat the High Cost of High Achievement_ (New York: Doubleday, 1980). Copyright © 1980 by Herbert J. Freudenberger, Ph.D. and Geraldine Richelson. Reprinted by permission of Doubleday, a division of Bantam, Doubleday, Dell Publishing Group, Inc.

onds) and then pick the number from the rating scale that represents the category which is most appropriate for you for that question.

Freudenberger advises that the higher the score, the more concern about the potential to develop cumulative stress there should be. But people should not be panicked because they can still do something about their stress level. The sooner a person starts taking care of himself or herself, the better. The next few chapters will be of great assistance in providing ideas about protecting oneself from and recovering from acute, delayed, and cumulative stress reactions.

SUMMARY

Recognition of the common signs and symptoms of acute and delayed stress reactions as well as those of Post Traumatic Stress Disorder (PTSD) is usually the first step in recovering from critical incident stress reactions. Change is one of the most important factors that indicates the presence of a stress reaction. Changes from a person's usual behavior should be noted, and every effort must be made to rebalance the person before the effects of stress become permanent. Critical incidents that produce acute and delayed reactions and may form the origins of PTSD are usually readily identifiable since the events that produce the stress reactions are dramatic and noticeable.

Cumulative stress reactions, on the other hand, are much slower to develop and much more subtle. They do not have the dramatic incident that starts them. They are made up of a mixture of personal and job-related problems which grow steadily worse over time. They are therefore more difficult to recognize and are also more difficult to cure.

In the remaining chapters we present many suggestions that will assist emergency personnel in mitigating and resolving acute, delayed, and cumulative stress reactions.

REFERENCES

1. *Webster's Seventh New Collegiate Dictionary.* (1965). Springfield, MA: G. & C. Merriam.
2. Pelletier, K. R. (1977). *Mind as Healer, Mind as Slayer: A Holistic Approach to Preventing Stress Disorders.* New York: Delta Books.
3. Mitchell, J. T. (1982). Recovery from rescue. *Response,* Fall, 7–10.
4. Mitchell, J. T. (1986). Critical incident stress management. *Response,* Sept./ Oct., 24–25.
5. Selye, H. (1982). History and present status of the stress concept. In L. Goldberger and S. Breznitz (Eds.), *Handbook of Stress: Theoretical and Clinical Aspects.* New York: Free Press, pp. 7–17.
6. Horowitz, M. J. (1986). *Stress Response Syndromes.* Northvale, NJ: Jason Aronson.
7. Adams, J. D. (1980). *Understanding and Managing Stress: A Book of Readings.* La Jolla, CA: University Associates.
8. Gherman, E. M. (1981). *Stress and the Bottom Line, a Guide to Personal Well-Being and Corporate Health.* New York: AMACOM.
9. Numerof, R. E. (1983). *Managing Stress: A Guide for Health Professionals.* Rockville, MD: Aspen Systems Corporation.

10. Girdano, D. A., and Everly, G. S. (1986). *Controlling Stress and Tension: A Holistic Approach.* Englewood Cliffs, NJ: Prentice-Hall.

11. Brallier, L. (1982). *Successfully Managing Stress.* Los Altos, CA: National Nursing Review.

12. Appelbaum, S. H. (1981). *Stress Management for Health Care Professionals.* Rockville, MD: Aspen Systems Corporation.

13. Everly, G. S., and Girdano, D. A. (1980). *The Stress Mess Solution.* Bowie, MD: R. J. Brady Co.

14. Flynn, P. A. (1980). *Holistic Health, the Art and Science of Care.* Bowie, MD: R. J. Brady Co.

15. Schneider, J. (1984). *Stress, Loss and Grief.* Baltimore: University Park Press.

16. Everly, G. S., and Sobelman (1987). *Assessment of the Human Stress Response.* New York: AMS Press.

17. van der Kolk, B. A. (Ed.). (1984). *Post Traumatic Stress Disorder: Psychological and Biological Sequelae.* Washington, DC: American Psychiatric Press.

18. Everly, G. S. (1989). *A Clinical Guide to the Treatment of Human Stress.* New York: Plenum.

19. van der Kolk, B. A. (1987). *Psychological Trauma.* Washington, DC: American Psychiatric Press.

20. Hartsough, D. M., and Garaventa Myers, D. (1985). Effects of stress on disaster workers. In D. M. Hartsough and D. Garaventa Myers, Eds., *Disaster Work and Mental Health: Prevention and Control of Stress among Workers.* Rockville, MD: Center for Mental Health Studies of Emergencies, U. S. Department of Health and Human Services.

21. Kroes, W. H., and Hurrell, J. J. (Eds.). (1975). *Job Stress and the Police Officer: Identifying Stress Reduction Techniques: Proceedings of Symposium.* Washington, DC: U.S. Government Printing Office.

22. Mitchell, J. T. (1986). By their own hand: Suicide among emergency workers. *Chief Fire Executive, 2*(1), 48–52; 65; 72.

23. Cooper, C. L. (1981). *Executive Families under Stress.* Englewood Cliffs, NJ: Prentice-Hall.

24. Cox,T. (1978). *Stress.* Baltimore: University Park Press.

25. Mitchell, J. T. (1985). Healing the helper. In Green, B. (Ed.). *Role Stressors and Supports for Emergency Workers.* Washington, DC: Center for Mental Health Studies of Emergencies, U.S. Department of Health and Human Services.

26. Scrignar, C. B. (1984). *Post Traumatic Stress Disorder: Diagnosis, Treatment, and Legal Issues.* New York: Praeger.

27. American Psychiatric Association. (1987). Post-traumatic stress disorder. *Diagnostic and Statistical Manual of Mental Disorders,* 3rd ed., rev. (DSM-III-R). Washington, DC: APA.

28. Edelwich, J. (1980). *Burn-Out: Stages of Disillusionment in the Helping Professions*. New York: Human Sciences Press.

29. Mitchell, J. T. (1981). *Emergency Response to Crisis*. Bowie, MD: R. J. Brady Co.

30. Farber, B. A. (Ed.). (1983). *Stress and Burnout in Human Service Professions*. Elmsford, NY: Pergamon Press.

31. Patrick, P. K. (1981). *Health Care Worker Burnout: What It Is, What to Do about It*. Chicago: Inquiry Books.

32. Hurrell, J. J., Pate, A., and Kliesmet, R. (1984). *Stress among Police Officers*. Washington, DC: National Institute for Occupational Safety and Health, U.S. Department of Health and Human Services.

33. Jones, J. (Ed.). (1981). *The Burnout Syndrome: Current Research, Theory, Interventions*. Park Ridge, IL: London House Press.

4

STRESS SURVIVAL SKILLS

Tones sound. An alarm is heard and suddenly emergency responders experience a pronounced shift from low to high activity levels. During this transition their focus of attention is directed to the external world and the problems inherent in an emergency response. Little time or attention is allocated for processing the multiple internal changes associated with their stress. This lack of awareness can lead to significant problems during either routine or critical situations. In this chapter we present specific skills and techniques that will enable responders to survive and master the stressful rigors of emergency response.

SURVIVING THE SHORT RESPONSE

Survival during the emergency incident, which lasts only a short time, depends heavily on the preincident training. Most emergency personnel function on "autopilot" during an incident that consumes only a short amount of time. Significant stress reactions can be reduced or eliminated if personnel are well trained and properly equipped to perform at a maximum level. They should not only be given the technical skills necessary to prepare them to perform under stressful conditions, but should also be given sufficient "human elements" training, such as crisis intervention and stress management training, so that they know how to help others in a state of acute emotional distress. They should also be aware of their own vulnerabilities to acute stress reactions and know the signs and symptoms of distress in themselves (see Chapter 3 for additional information).

Proper eating habits, the right foods and a regular exercise program to maintain proper physical fitness help to keep emergency personnel ready to perform their jobs even under the worst possible conditions. It is foolish to expect that people can spring into action without endangering themselves when they have not put time and effort into maintaining themselves before the emergency.

During an incident leadership should be decisive, effective, and efficient. This, of course, is impossible to achieve if leaders refuse to accept intensive training and if they have not drilled extensively with their crews prior to the crisis event. Good leadership does not appear suddenly at a scene. It is built over a long period of time after the expenditure of considerable energy and a willingness to learn from mistakes and absorb new, effective ideas.

Emergency workers are urged to follow the legitimate commands of well-trained, experienced, knowledgeable leaders. Their physical and emotional well-being is frequently in the hands of their leadership. An effective emergency response relies on an open communication and a flowing interaction between their leaders and themselves.

New members of an emergency team should not be placed in the most precarious situations during an emergency. Instead, they should work with well-trained and experienced personnel who can teach them the tricks of field survival without endangering them. Accepting the supervision of those with greater experience is an important survival strategy.

As much information about the emergency event as possible should be passed off from the dispatcher to the field responders. Updates of information in route should be given whenever possible. The less surprising the incident, the less likelihood there is that emergency personnel will be affected by it negatively.

Personnel should do their best to manage the incident. However, they should be careful not to take on personal blame for the occurrence of the incident. It happened before they arrived and they cannot lose valuable energy trying to find a way to blame themselves for the event. Emergency personnel do not cause the tragedies to which they respond. They simply have the training, the drive, and the experience to do whatever they can to intervene in the midst of a chaotic occurrence.

Immediately after an event, the unit is restored to a state of readiness. At that time all team members should take a little care of themselves. That care can come in the form of a shower, a half-hour rest period followed by a meal, or physical exercise to burn off some of the harmful chemicals associated with a stress response. Personnel would be wise to avoid or limit their intake of caffeine products and sugar. Fluid replacement is very important. However, alcohol is to be avoided absolutely. Alcohol is contraindicated as a stress control method because it makes the stress response in the body and the mind far more powerful than it should be. Similarly, other substance abuse methods of dealing with stress reactions are extremely dangerous to the health and well-being of emergency personnel.[1,2]

Emergency workers are urged to talk about a bad incident with trusted friends. Talking helps to clear one's mind about the incident and put things in perspective. It frequently helps them to understand that the incident is bothering a number of people. They feel less alone and less abnormal.

Feedback (both positive and negative, which is presented as a learning strategy) is important for emergency workers. They need to know when and how a not-so-good job was done and what can be done by them to correct their mistakes. But most especially, they need to know when they did a good job and that their efforts are appreciated.

They may benefit from a psychological debriefing, called a Critical Incident Stress Debriefing (CISD) when an event has been particularly distressing. More will be said about the CISD process in Chapters 5 and 7.

SURVIVAL DURING A PROLONGED EMERGENCY RESPONSE

Time Orientation

Our sense of time evolves out of years of experience. As a child, "two weeks until Christmas" seemed like an eternity. As we age, our frame of reference expands and life events give a different perspective to time. As adults, two weeks can feel like a very short time. In a critical or highly stressful situation, the time frame is again altered. A responder may lose track of time with no apparent awareness that many minutes or even hours have passed since a response started. This lack of awareness can lead to significant problems during field operations. Fatigue builds, physical and emotional efficiency decreases, and there is increased risk for mistakes or injuries.

Regular time reorientation for all responding team members is an effective way to increase their internal monitoring of physical, mental, and emotional reserves. The reorientation can be handled by a supervisor, team leader, or team member. It is sufficient for the person to identify current time and elapsed time since arrival on the scene. Twenty-minute intervals between time announcements are appropriate. A commander or some other member of the response group should remind the personnel of the current and elapsed times. An occasional announcement about times over the loudspeakers of emergency apparatus can be helpful as long as it is not interfering with other important field communications.

Rest/Rotation

As responders monitor internal reserves more effectively, the need for appropriate rest periods will become more apparent. Prolonged responses require a more efficient use of resources. Rest periods enable a response team to function for a much longer total period of time. Short-term responses obviously require less attention to reserves or time flow. Responses greater than two hours in duration should alert command personnel to the need for possible intervention and alterations in operational procedures.

A good rule of thumb to follow in field operations is to provide 30 minutes of rest after every two-hour period of stressful work. *Two hours on, then 30 minutes of downtime.* This rest/work schedule can be followed for twelve hours at the scene. *Twelve-hour maximum time limits at the scene should be the goal.* Most people make more mistakes or get injured more frequently when they have just spent twelve hours doing something, regardless of what it is.

Call in additional help. Help should be requested before the first rest period. Why risk mistakes and injuries with fatigued people? Fresh personnel add energy and open minds to the critical work of emergency services. Often, their new ideas help to improve the speed and efficiency of the operation.

In some instances, the stress at a scene will be so intense that some emergency personnel may not be able to work a full two hours before they are given a break. Special accommodations must be made for personnel who have been hit with an extraordinary stress. The first step is to cut down on their exposure to the sights, sounds, and smells of the immediate scene. Remove them a short distance away and have a peer support person stay with them until their vital signs can be monitored and the command staff and the medical officer are assured that the person's stress reaction is not so severe as to become life threatening (stress when ignored may produce cardiac arrythmias and possibly cardiac arrest).[3] Then the person should be given some rest (about fifteen minutes) before any decisions are made to return the person to service. If the person's physical and emotional condition improves and is able to go back in service, it is advisable that he or she be reassigned to a different task so as not to be in danger of developing another reaction to the same stimuli.

Occasionally, some emergency service personnel are especially badly hit by a critical incident. Finding the dead body of a close friend who was killed in action is an example of something that could completely overwhelm one's coping abilities. They may be overcome by powerful emotions beyond their usual ability to deal with a bad situation. The emotional impact is so powerful that the person cannot function adequately at the scene. This reaction is a *normal reaction* of a *normal person* to a totally *abnormal event.*

If a responder to an awful incident experiences such a powerful emotional reaction that he or she is unable to function adequately at the scene, and if rest and a cutting of the adverse stimuli is not sufficient to restore them to at least a minimally acceptable level of performance, it may be necessary to extend their rest break substantially. At times, a commanding officer might have to consider removal from the scene to a quiet place, another emergency services facility such as a fire station or a police station, or to a hospital if medical evaluation appears necessary. *Removal of seriously distressed personnel from the scene is not the first stress control method that should be initiated.* It is utilized only when other appropriate methods have failed to restore the distressed crew members to an acceptable level of function.[4]

In some extraordinary circumstances, evacuation to one's home may be necessary. This is a *last resort* decision. If a decision is made to remove a team member to his or her home, the family members should be called and informed of the situation and the reasons for the decision to remove the worker. One or two members of the distressed workers organization should accompany the individual to his or her home and remain with the family and the distressed person until the intense reaction subsides. Calling in a peer or professional support person from a CISD team to assist a highly stressed emergency responder is a wise move. These trained people do much to reduce stress for the affected person. The idea is to place the distressed person in a situation in which a family member or a trained support person is alerted to the distress so that the proper support can be provided. If no one is home, the decision to remove the person from the scene must be altered. Instead of sending the distressed person home, the command staff would be better to choose a fire or police station or other place where there are emergency personnel. The main idea is to make sure that the distressed person is not left completely alone. However, it is also important to make sure that people are not hovering over a distressed person. They need some breathing space. People should be available to them but not hovering over them. Shutting down station house operations may be necessary. Cut radio traffic, telephones, tones, and so on. Have other units handle the calls.

Normally emergency crews are removed or replaced as total units. That is, they arrive at the scene together and are disengaged from action or from the scene together. The wise incident commander calls for help early in the incident before the crews become fatigued. In that way, fresh personnel will be available for crew rotation. In most cases pulling out only a part of a working crew is disruptive to the team cohesiveness.

In a circumstance in which the scene is so severely confined that only a few people can work at a task, a team that normally works together should relieve its own members by subdividing into smaller subgroups. In such circumstances, commanders should also attempt to change only a portion of the work crew at a time by bringing in a few fresh personnel to replace those most exhausted. Later, other fresh workers can be added to the work crew as the remaining tired team members are removed to lighter assignments or to the rest area. Also, the new crew leader comes inside the internal perimeter to monitor the phased change of crews, to observe the operation, make suggestions, and receive a briefing from the leader who has led the operation to this point. The leader who is about to be relieved stays inside the perimeter until the full change of crews is accomplished and the operation is handed off to the new crew leader.

It is also extremely important to keep the crew supervisors with the crews. People become far more stressed when they feel that they have absent leadership. They experience the increased pressure of having to make all of the decisions without the benefit of the leader's knowledge and proper support.

A word of caution regarding the resting of teams working at an emergency. Emergency personnel will experience frustration and anger if they are rested too often or before it is necessary for them to take a break. For example, if they are required to take a break every 20 minutes, they will generally feel that the rest breaks are interfering with their ability to do their jobs properly.

Similarly, rest breaks that are forced upon emergency workers who are only a very few minutes from completion of their mission will cause frustration, anger, and far more stress than if they had been able to complete their job. Appropriate rest breaks are very important for all emergency workers. However, the rest breaks must be carefully timed and necessary if they are to be effective in reducing stress. Rest breaks should help people to do their jobs—*not* increase their stress.

In most cases, the greatest effectiveness can be achieved when reassignment to a rest area is not abrupt. If possible, the person on the front line should be moved to a less intense work area for a while before being sent to a rest area. In other words, a graduated decrease in activity is much better than a total change from full activity to no activity.

Whenever possible, emergency personnel should be sent to lighter-duty work stations before going to intensely stressful work areas. This staging strategy also allows time for fresh people to orient themselves to the situation before becoming fully responsible for the critical activities.

People should be told that they will be given a break within a certain time range so that they are not surprised when they are taken off the front line. If policies regarding rest can be established in advance for emergency personnel, they will accept rest breaks as a normal procedure and will not feel that they are being punished or unfairly singled out when told to take a break. Figure 4–1 illustrates a model for the rotation of crews.

When it is not possible to rotate personnel to full rest status because the incident is so big that it requires all of the available team members, a secondary strategy of reassigning people is important. Prolonged exposure to a limited scope of work can be decreased by reassigning workers to different tasks. Reassignment enables the person to break out of the tunnel vision which often accompanies prolonged tension-filled activity around the same task.

It should be noted that command officers have a responsibility to take breaks themselves. Their personnel rely on their ability to make sound decisions. Failure to follow the rest policies discussed in this chapter and elsewhere exposes commanders to the same stress reactions encountered by their personnel. It also makes them less efficient in their leadership. A mistake made by a fatigued leader who has failed to rest properly in a reasonable manner may produce serious injury or even death to an emergency worker. That type of irresponsible behavior may actually make a command officer open to personal legal liabilities in today's lawsuit-prone society.

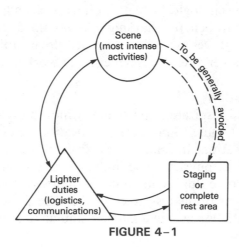

FIGURE 4–1

Physiological Considerations

Shelter

Human behavior can be significantly changed by exposure to cold, heat, altitude, and dehydration. These factors also reduce the ability of people to deal with stress.[5-7] Provision of appropriate shelter is a high priority in a prolonged situation, especially in foul weather. School buildings, community centers, union halls, houses of worship, and tents all make good shelters. Ambulances and large enclosed rescue vehicles may serve as good temporary rest stations. Whenever possible these facilities should be equipped with chairs and/or cots. *Keep people warm and dry when they are not involved at the scene.*

Toilet Facilities

Prolonged field activity can also alter basic physical responses, including hydration and waste elimination. As described in the section on physical response to stress, the digestive system can be strongly affected by stress. A frequent response to nervousness or tension is an increase in bowel secretion, leading to diarrhea.[8]

During prolonged field operations adequate plans should be enacted to address the increased need for portable toilet facilities. Effective planners will also anticipate that the standard number of rolls of tissue allocated to a portable toilet will be insufficient for a prolonged emergency situation since most companies base allocations of supplies on normal, not highly stressed, work-site situations.

Portable wash sinks are an imporant feature of a well-run field operation. This is especially true if people are involved in body recovery operations. The psychological benefit of having clean hands far surpasses almost any other health benefits that might be obtained. Similarly, having a supply of clean work gloves available to replace gloves soiled with blood, feces, and body pieces is very helpful to emergency workers.

Rehydration

Increased respiration (particularly mouth breathing), perspiration, and urination contribute to possible dehydration associated with prolonged situations. Alterations in fluid and electrolyte balance can strongly affect cognitive as well as physical functioning. Unfortunately, most attempts at rehydration involve fluids containing caffeine. Caffeine is a chemical that can make the effects of distress much worse. The choice to use fluids containing caffeine should be made in a manner similar to a physician prescribing medication.[9]

When is the most advantageous time for the use of caffeine? When, in an incident, would tired emergency responders derive the maximum benefit from the "lift" associated with caffeine? The best answer requires a good analysis of the situation and the personnel involved. Generally, serious fatigue begins four to six hours (as observed by the authors) into most responses. If the use of caffeinated beverages could be delayed for at least four hours, personnel would gain the best physiological benefit from them.

Each person should be cautious in using caffeine products. Both past studies as well as research currently under way suggest that caffeine can have significant negative side effects even at low levels and should not exceed reasonable levels of consumption.[10] It is possible that the presence of caffeine in one's system during a critical incident may heighten the chance of developing Post Traumatic Stress Disorder (see Chapters 2 and 3) or make the disorder worse should it occur. Coffee, tea, and cola drinks all contain caffeine, which contributes to the dehydration of the body. *Be cautious with caffeine.*

Alcohol is absolutely inappropriate during and for a considerable period of time after the emergency. It directly increases stress reactions and causes problems with judgment, decision making, and behavior. Alcohol significantly increases the danger of legal liabilities for all emergency workers involved in an incident. It will also directly enhance dehydration in those who utilize it.[11]

Soda also has hazards. Besides the fact that it is loaded with sugar, most sodas have a great deal of phosphorus. Too much phosphorus disrupts the body's calcium/phosphorus balance. Disruptions in the calcium/phosphorus balance set the stage for potential development of kidney stones and bone diseases. *Go easy on soft drinks.*

It is recommended that plenty of water and fruit juices or specially formulated soft drinks (diluted by at least one-fourth or one-half to avoid "sugar shock") be utilized for the first four hours before caffeine products are introduced. *The use of special thirst quenchers has a hidden danger.* Commercially available thirst quenchers tend to suppress the natural body signals that cause a person to drink more water. As a result, some people may not think that they need water when they actually need much more than they are consuming. *Cool water is the best rehydration agent.*[12]

Some people still think that salt tablets are effective in reducing the chance of dehydration. *The use of salt tablets should be discouraged.* Salt tablets have been known to produce sodium chloride toxicity in some cases. It is more likely that the concentrated salt in the tablet will cause stomach-lining irritation. Concentrated salt may cause the stomach lining to bleed and may slow absorbtion of water into the body system from the small and large intestines. In fact, salt may draw water into the stomach from the body, thus depriving the muscles of the water they need to function properly. Cramps may also result if water is drawn into the stomach. *Salt tablets may be the worst choice for hard-working personnel facing the potential of dehydration.* The availability of an adequate supply of water is a far better solution to the dehydration problem.[12]

Food

Food for personnel involved in a prolonged field mission is also of considerable concern. To keep active personnel functioning at their very best, the right kinds of foods need to be provided at the scene. Emergency workers need virtually none of the sugar or fat-loaded foods they are frequently given in the field. The usual field diet consists of hot dogs, hamburgers, sugar donuts, candy bars, cookies, and pastries, which are washed down with large volumes of soda and coffee. Sugar increases the potential that emergency personnel are going to be irritable, hyperactive, and eventually depressed. Sugar in the stomach will draw water into the stomach from the muscles and other parts of the body. The end result may be cramps and muscle dehydration.

Fats cannot provide the fuel necessary to carry emergency personnel through the spurts of intensely strenuous activity at the scene. It takes oxygen to break fats down into usable body fuel. Oxygen is not as available for the breakdown of fat during brief spurts of activity as it is when the body is involved in consistent exercise. Only if the exercise activity becomes consistent over 20 minutes or more does oxygen enter the bloodstream in sufficient levels to begin to assist the liver in breaking down the fat. Even under circumstances of consistent aerobic exercise, fat is more difficult to break down into glycogen (stored fuel in the liver) and eventually the body's fuel, glucose (usable fuel in the bloodstream), than are complex carbohydrates. The entire process of breaking fat down into glycogen may take as long as 90 minutes. Obviously, fat is not a good source of readily available energy. Instead, it usually sits in the stomach or intestines, gives the worker a heavy, too-full feeling, and takes up the space that might better be given to the more efficient complex carbohydrates. This irrational diet is not in the best interests of the field responder and causes physical stress.[12,13]

Some people believe that the proteins in meats are a requisite for emergency personnel in the field. This is not necessarily true. Americans eat far too much protein in their everyday diet. Proteins are necessary for the body, but they are a poor source of immediate energy. *Complex carbohydrates are*

TABLE 4–1   Foods for Emergencies

FOOD	BENEFIT
Plain granola bars	Complex carbohydrates
Fruits (fresh)	Carbohydrates and fiber (some vitamins)
Fruits (dried)	Carbohydrates and fiber (ease of storage)
Milk	Proteins and calcium
Hard cheeses	Proteins and calcium
Whole-grain breads	Complex carbohydrates
Crackers	Complex carbohydrates
Fresh vegetables	Complex carbohydrates (vitamins)

a far better source of energy than are proteins or fats. It is generally not necessary to be overly concerned about protein intake during a mission because the average responder comes to the scene with more than enough protein in his or her system to carry the worker through the field operation. What is recommended instead is a good nutritious meal after a period of rest (or about 30 minutes) at the conclusion of the incident. A good meal after the incident will usually restore the depleted proteins. In Table 4–1 we suggest the best foods for supporting emergency personnel through a prolonged field operation.[12,14]

Eliminating Surprises

One of the most devastating factors for emergency personnel working during field emergencies is the element of surprise. Surprises tend to catch people off guard. Before they are able to continue their work, surprised personnel must gain control of the feelings of shock and denial which are generated by surprise. The only emergency workers who should be the victims of surprise are the first arrivals, who get thrown into the situation with little warning. It is not necessary for the later-arriving crews to be caught off guard simply because their predecessors could not be given adequate information about what faced them.

Providing pre-deployment briefings to all new arrivals at a scene helps to cut down on the amount and intensity of surprises among emergency personnel. Telling responders what they are about to face helps them to get used to the idea intellectually before they have to face it in reality. For example, if you tell an emergency worker that a victim has been decapitated, the worker has time to deal intellectually with the victim's condition before having to face the sight itself.

Mission Clarification

A briefing upon arrival at an emergency situation helps a person clarify the nature of the event and assists personnel in establishing a preplan of activity. This cuts down on job ambiguity and confusion. It helps the emergency worker to know exactly what is expected. Additionally, clarification of the leadership is also possible during the preaction briefing. When emergency personnel know who is in charge, they experience less confusion and are more effective and efficient in the performance of their duties.

When new information becomes available during the incident, working crews should have the benefit of the new knowledge. New information helps people adjust to the changes in the demands upon them and makes them feel as though the command staff has interest in their welfare.

Feedback is essential. Emergency personnel need to know how they are doing and whether their efforts are paying off. Encouragement and appreciation are important for fatigued personnel. *"Thank you" goes a long way.*

Deployment

Once people have been informed of the particulars of the incident and a decision is made to utilize certain resources, rapid deployment of the personnel is necessary. Unnecessary waiting at the scene intensifies stress reactions by heightening anxiety and boredom. *Evaluate, Decide, Inform, Deploy!*

Stimuli Reduction

When emergency people are given the opportunity to rest, they should be removed from auditory, olfactory, and visual stimuli. Studies show that exposure to gory sights and sometimes repulsive odors and sounds associated with emergency work may intensify and continue acute stress reactions. For instance, noises in the range 2000 to 4000 hertz are considered most capable of producing strong physiological stress reactions in average human beings. Human screams rate just about 3000 hertz on the scale. They are quite capable of producing significant physical responses in emergency people who are exposed to them.[15]

A quiet place with little or no aversive auditory and visual stimuli is the best circumstance for resting emergency crews. At the very least, resting crews should be facing away from the scene and should not be listening to operational radio traffic during their rest breaks. Hearing and vision protection is also essential in reducing stress-producing stimuli. Good leaders always insist on maximum protection of the health and well being of their personnel.

Physical Exercise

The human stress response has been designed for an intense level of physical activity. Strenuous physical work during an incident may actually be helpful in reducing the overall impact of psychological stress. Of course, excessive physical exertion leads to fatigue and a variety of physical and psychological aftereffects. Most injuries occur when emergency personnel are fatigued. A balance between hard work and appropriate rest periods is highly encouraged.[5]

After an emergency is completed, crew members will gain considerable benefit from participation in strenuous physical exercise. (Of course, it is assumed that personnel are physically able to perform physical exercise and that they have been cleared by their physician for such activity.) Physical exercise must take place within 24 hours of a stressful event or it will not be as beneficial in reducing the level of harmful stress reactions in the body. The closer the physical exercise is to the time of the incident, the better. The longer the time frame from the impact of the event, the less benefit is the physical exercise. *Utilize physical exertion exercise shortly after a stressful situation to reduce the overall level of harmful stress chemicals in the body.*[1,12,16]

Physical exercise burns off the high levels of stress chemicals that accumulate in the body during a stress-filled incident. The chemicals of stress reactions are quite caustic and deteriorate body cells. Utilizing physical exercise as a stress reduction strategy helps to balance out the body's chemical reaction and returns body chemicals to more normal levels. When a person cannot sleep after a distressing call, physical exercise may help to calm the system and enhance the opportunities for better rest.[12,17] The best exercise for stress reduction is aerobic exercise. Running, swimming, fast walking, tennis, racquet ball, and volleyball are among the activities that seem to have the best benefit.

Safety

When emergency personnel are preoccupied with a scene, they may be more careless about their own personal safety. Few have not looked back on some incident or another and thought "How could I have done that? That was dumb and dangerous!" To avoid or cut down the amount and seriousness of the injuries that an emergency team member encounters, personnel should develop the habit of *always* utilizing the proper protective gear. At any scene where special hazards exist, a safety officer should be appointed. This does not sound very elaborate as a stress management strategy. But sometimes the simplest stress strategies tend to be the best. *Safety should not be the concern of the leadership alone; it should be a concern for all responders to an incident.*

Prepare for the Unexpected

In some critical incidents, spouses and family members of dead or injured emergency service personnel have come to the scene to await word about their loved one. Personnel engaged in operations found this situation to be quite unnerving, for several reasons. First, they had information about the emergency personnel and could not share it with the family members. They felt that if the family members saw their faces they would know that there was bad news, so they looked away or, even worse, walked away from these family members of their fellow workers. They felt guilty and uncomfortable about their treatment of the family members but did not know what else to do.

Second, some of their own family members came to the scene because they were worried about their spouses or family members who were involved in the operation. Contact with one's own family at a scene stirs emotions that would normally not be present during a mission.

Provision should be made to have a chaplain or mental health professional and a ranking officer who is a caring person assigned as part of a family liaison team. Family members should be given accurate information about the situation and the condition of their loved one as soon as it becomes available. They should also be reasonably protected from seeing gory sights around the scene. It is frequently best to gather them in a building a short distance away from the scene.

A family liaison officer should also be sent to the hospital if unit members have been sent there because they have been injured. If the organization has a *Critical Incident Stress Debriefing Team* available, it should be called in to assist the families. Support services for family members should be provided as soon as possible and should be continued for a reasonable period of time after conclusion of the incident.

Many emergency workers in a major incident are extremely worried about their family members at home. Rules that prohibit brief phone calls home to reassure family members of the safety of the workers or to allow them to check on the well-being of their families may need to be suspended temporarily. In fact, in a major incident it would be extremely helpful if cellular phones could be brought in to assist emergency personnel in making brief contacts with their families. Both the families and the emergency workers will benefit and feel that they are supported and appreciated.

Media at the Scene

Emergency teams must expect an influx of members of the media, so a media liaison officer should be appointed. All personnel must be instructed to direct members of the media to that officer and not provide direct comments about the mission to media personnel.

It is important to remind emergency personnel that they do not have to talk to the media to be quoted. If they make a remark to a fellow worker and it is overheard by a media representative, they will be quoted even if their names do not appear in the report. This particular practice on the part of the media may therefore produce inaccurate or exaggerated reports that make emergency personnel look bad in the eyes of the public.

Signals of Distress

Emergency personnel can lessen feelings of guilt, shame, frustration, and anger by being fully aware of the stress symptoms they are likely to encounter under field conditions. For example, many police officers feel like cowards because they began to shake while under gun fire. If they knew that this was a *normal* physiological response to the presence of adrenalin in their body systems and not a sign of cowardice, they would feel less guilty about their shaking.

Knowledge becomes strength. The more emergency personnel know about stress before a crisis strikes, the better able they will be to deal with the incident.[18]

SUMMARY

In this chapter we reviewed a variety of helpful stress management strategies which are particularly useful during operations in the field. Methods of reducing, controlling, and eliminating stress in both the short-duration and prolonged events were presented. Emergency personnel were urged to be familiar with the common signs of distress so that they might be better prepared to assist fellow workers or recognize stress in themselves. It was also suggested that emergency personnel eat properly before the event and try to rest between calls. It was pointed out that well-trained personnel who are doing their best to manage an event should not attempt to accept personal blame for the tragedies they encounter in the field.

To enhance stress management in a prolonged incident, basic areas of field operations were addressed. They include:

- Time orientation
- Rest/rotation
- Physiological considerations

Commanders and front-line personnel were urged to make provision for, among other things, shelter, toilet facilities, rehydration of workers, food, and information flow to those working at the scene. The more human needs which are managed in the field, the less likelihood there is that stress will take an unnecessary toll on the emergency services.

REFERENCES

1. Gherman, E. M. (1981). *Stress and the Bottom Line.* New York: AMACOM.
2. Numerof, R. E. (1983). *Managing Stress: A Guide for Health Professional.* Rockville, MD: Aspen Systems Corporation.
3. Hafen, B. Q. (1981). *How to Live Longer: Practical Ways You Can Beat Stress, Heart Disease, Cancer, Infection and Chronic Illness.* Englewood Cliffs, NJ: Prentice-Hall.
4. Mitchell, J. T. (1983). When disaster strikes: The critical incident stress debriefing process. *Journal of Emergency Medical Services, 8*(1), 36–39.
5. Hockey, R., Ed. (1983). *Stress and Fatigue in Human Performance.* New York: Wiley.
6. Grant, H., et al. (1985). *Action Guide for Emergency Service Personnel.* Bowie, MD: Brady Communications Co.
7. Gazzaniga, A. B., Iseri, L. T., and Baren, M. (1982). *Emergency Care Principles and Practices for the EMT-Paramedic.* Reston, VA: Reston.
8. van der Kolk, B. A., Boyd, H., Krystal, J., and Greenberg, M. (1984). *Post Traumatic Stress Disorder: Psychological and Biological Sequelae.* Washington, DC: American Psychiatric Press.
9. Everly, G. S. and Rosenfeld, R. (1981). *The Nature and Treatment of the Stress Response: A Practical Guide for Clinicians.* New York: Plenum.
10. Brallier, L. (1982). *Successfully Managing Stress.* Los Altos, CA: National Nursing Review.
11. Monat, A., and Lazarus, R. (Eds.). (1985). *Stress and Coping: An Anthology.* (2nd Ed.). New York: Columbia University Press.
12. Matteson, M. T., and Ivancevich, J. M. (1982). *Managing Job Stress and Health.* New York: Free Press.
13. Flynn, P. A. R. (1980). *Holistic Health: The Art and Science of Care.* Bowie, MD: R. J. Brady Co.

14. Smith, S. (1988). Food for fast times. *America West Airlines Magazine, 2*(12): 79–82.

15. Stone, J. (1988). Triumph of the Willies. *Discovery, 9*(4): 80; 82–83.

16. Girdano, D. A. and Everly, G. S. (1986). *Controlling Stress Tension: A Holistic Approach.* (2nd Ed.). Englewood Cliffs, NJ: Prentice-Hall.

17. Pelletier, K. R. (1977). *Mind as Healer, Mind as Slayer: A Holistic Approach to Preventing Stress Disorders.* New York: Delta Books.

18. Ayoob, M. F. (1984). Stress Fire. *Gun Fighting for Police: Advanced Tactics and Techniques.* Concord, NH: Police Bookshelf Publishers.

5

ORGANIZATION-SPONSORED STRESS SURVIVAL SKILLS

In Chapter 4 we developed some ideas for stress control during short or prolonged emergency incidents. In this chapter we go beyond Chapter 4 and suggest a number of things that can be done at the organizational level before crisis events strike. What will be emphasized in this chapter are policy issues, procedures, and programs that can be planned for, developed, and implemented without the pressures associated with an emergency response. The strategies discussed in this chapter will enhance the emergency responder's ability to cope effectively with stress both during the emergency incident and during the more routine happenings of everyday emergency services life.

SCREENING

There is a job/personality match that people need to accommodate in their lives. If the job and the personality do not complement each other, frustration and unhappiness result. This is especially so in the emergency services. The jobs of emergency services personnel are very specialized and demand a very special personality (see Chapter 2).

Sometimes the wrong types of people manage to get into emergency work. They do not have the right personality or they may have the wrong motivation for getting into the work. They end up failing at the job or becoming very unhappy people as they make attempts to succeed. Sometimes they turn their frustrations on their fellow workers or, even worse, on the people they are supposed to serve. They make themselves and everyone around them miserable with their chronic complaints, irritability, and continuous battles with commanders over relatively insignificant problems. Cumulative stress problems increase for them and everyone wishes they would just go away.

In recent years considerable progress has been made in developing better screening procedures for emergency service personnel. The selection processes often include several of the following items:[1-4]

- Written applications
- Written tests
- Personal interview(s)
- Assessment stations
- Physical agility and stamina tests
- Psychological test batteries
- Committee interviews
- Videotaped interview sessions
- Background checks for criminal or psychiatric problems
- Medical evaluations
- Follow-up on references and prior jobs
- Psychological interviews
- Team worker evaluations
- Probationary periods
- Etc.

Despite these and other measures, it is not always possible to predict accurately who will do well or badly in emergency work. However, performing a number of the evaluation techniques above should give the commanders of emergency service units some reassurance that their choices are the best that can be made. (It is important to note that even volunteer organizations have a duty and an obligation to screen their personnel carefully. Screening protects citizens from poor performances by emergency services personnel and also protects the organization from the legal ramifications of inadequate screening.) *Choose the best!*

Organizations and command staff should make every possible effort to assure that the best possible job/personality match exists in personnel who are applying for positions in an emergency organization. This will reduce stress both within the organization and within the people who are chosen to work in it.

TECHNICAL SKILLS TRAINING

Stress can be prevented by means of education and training. People need to know how best to perform their jobs. They also need to know their capabilities and limitations. Knowing the technical aspects of their job makes them more self-reliant and confident. Knowledge and training eventually become good habits that make the knowledgeable person perform better under pressure.

Once the basic training is completed, emergency personnel need continuous training to keep their skills fresh and ready for application. Repetitive drills help the personnel know each other's abilities and reactions under pressure. The crews become teams and know better what to expect from one another. Commanders would be wise to drill with their personnel at least occasionally so that they, too, can become part of the team. Personnel know how best to work with the commanders when they see them in action—and vice versa, the commanders know how best to work with their personnel when they have practiced together. *Training builds teams.*

"HUMAN ELEMENTS" TRAINING

Few emergency personnel have been trained adequately to deal with the emotionally demanding events they must manage in their day-to-day work. They are asked to perform a great many skills for which they have received excellent technical training. They can usually accomplish these with little or no difficulty. However, when it comes to recognizing and appropriately intervening in situations in which other human beings are emotionally distressed, emergency workers are at a loss. They have never been taught crisis intervention skills. They are totally unsure of what to do to alleviate the emotional pain of another person. Only the basics of crisis intervention skills are taught to police officers and prehospital emergency medical personnel. Firefighters receive virtually no training in crisis intervention.

To alleviate this stress producing lack of knowledge, provision should be made to utilize existing materials or to develop new materials to teach police officers, emergency medical personnel, dispatchers, and firefighters how to assist distressed human beings more appropriately during crisis events. They should also be taught how to distinguish between those who are having a normal stress reaction during a crisis and those who are truly mentally disturbed.[5,6]

Having these courses taught before a crisis event can help to reduce the feelings of uncertainty and frustration that are stirred up in emergency personnel who are suddenly faced with distressed people in the midst of a crisis. Recruit personnel should be given an overview of crisis intervention skills before they graduate from academies. Knowing what to do under such circumstances or at least having a set of general guidelines is important because it lowers anxiety and increases the confidence of the responders.

Knowing what to do for another person is very important. However, educational efforts should not stop there. If the concepts presented in this book could be taught to emergency personnel before crisis events, emergency providers would be far better prepared to prevent serious stress reactions in themselves and their fellow workers. Add a stress management course to the recruit class requirements. The more knowledgeable personnel are about stress, the better able they are to assess stress reactions and intervene quickly with CISDs and other forms of support before excessive damage is done.[7]

Human elements training should include (but not be limited to) such topics as:[8]

- Crisis intervention skills
- Stress management skills
- Conflict resolution skills
- Human communications
- Behavioral emergencies
- Peer support services
- Disaster psychology
- Problem-solving skills
- Managing violent patients
- Assisting families of the dead

SUPERVISORY SKILLS

Traditionally in the emergency services, officers have been chosen from those who have progressed up through the ranks. Unfortunately, field experience does not necessarily guarantee management skills. Many emergency leaders have little or no management training to assist them in the performance of their jobs. They also lack some of the "people skills" which are so necessary to them to perform their jobs as supervisors and administrators. This situation produces stress for both the leaders and for those who are led.

Organizations have a responsibility to their command staff to make appropriate management training available to them before and after they assume their supervisory or management roles. The technical aspects of the job are important, of course, but so are the management issues. Supervisors must be made more aware of the clues to the performance abilities of their personnel. They should be aware of stress and the problems encountered because of it. Supervisors need improved human communication skills and knowledge about conflict resolution. There are many programs that will help supervisory personnel function better.[9]

Supervisors should take every step to assure themselves that they have adequate training. They should not balk at the chance to take courses and workshops designed to help them perform better in their roles. The philosophy should be: "If I can learn one new idea at a workshop that helps me be a better leader, it is worth it."

IMPROVED MANAGEMENT STYLES

Today leadership needs to approach its staff with a somewhat different approach from that which worked many years ago. The leadership styles that worked many years ago do not work today, for a number of reasons. First, the personnel themselves are better educated and have received a good deal of new and sophisticated technical training. Second, they have frequently not passed through strict military-style discipline and react quite differently to their commanders than do ex-military personnel. Third, emergency services people have been encouraged by programs like the incident command system to work together with their commanders in an interactive leadership. Under the incident command system, it must be recognized that rank does not provide anyone with a monopoly on good ideas. *Even the lowest-ranking person may sometimes have a good idea that is worth putting into practice.*[10]

PHYSICAL TRAINING

More detail regarding physical exercise is presented in Chapter 6. What is important to mention here is that it is important to have a policy toward physical training. Minimum levels of physical training should be established for each emergency organization. This is not something to be totally freelanced by each person. People need freedom to engage in whatever physical exercises are suitable for them. But they should be offered guidelines, education, and coaching so that they are able to stay in top condition. The recommendations in Chapter 6 call for aerobic exercise for 20 minutes three times a week and achieves a cardiac rate that is at least 70 percent of maximum heart rate. These standards may need to be adapted to the needs of a particular organization, and some flexibility must be maintained to allow for individual circumstances. The important thing is that there is a policy in the organization for physical training to help maintain the overall health and minimum fitness levels of the personnel.[11]

PREPLANNED MENTAL HEALTH SERVICES

Employee Assistance Programs

Emergency organizations across the nation are coming to the realization that it is more costly to replace personnel than to spend some money on programs to keep good personnel healthy, functioning, and on the job. They are also realizing that some employees are in such deep trouble that they need help in stabilizing themselves and getting relief from their problems. That is why *employee assistance programs* (EAPs) have been developed. They are particularly helpful for employees with alcohol and substance abuse problems, but many of them go much further and help employees with family problems, legal difficulties, and individual counseling. They are frequently a good source for referrals to other professionals.

Employee assistance programs are not miracle workers, however. It is especially difficult to help successfully an employee who has waited too long to come in for help. Early referrals are extremely important. It is also important to recognize that EAPs may have significant limitations. For example, since EAP groups are hired by the administration of a department, they may be viewed as an extension of administration and they have to work harder and very carefully to gain the trust of personnel. With some exceptions it has been found that EAPs are usually *not* the best group to coordinate Critical Incident Stress Debriefing (CISD) teams because the duties and procedures of an EAP do not necessarily blend with the duties and procedures of a CISD team.

Critical Incident Stress Debriefing Teams

Since 1974, a new approach to support personnel exposed to extremely distressing critical incidents has been developed and disseminated across the nation. The Critical Incident Stress Debriefing Team concept has been implemented in many communities and many more teams are in the planning stages.

The Critical Incident Stress Debriefing (CISD) is based on a partnership between mental health professionals and peer support personnel. Mental health professionals provide the special knowledge that is important in group facilitation, diagnosis of serious stress reactions which may need a little more help to resolve, and the education and supervision of peer support personnel. Peer support personnel have the ability to get close to emergency workers and are usually the first to see problems developing. Often peers, who utilize a well-trained but low-keyed approach to their fellow workers, are able to provide good-quality support at a place and time when no mental professionals are available.[12]

Critical Incident Stress Debriefing teams provide at least ten basic types of services. They are:

- Pre-incident stress training to all personnel
- On-scene support to obviously distressed personnel
- Individual consults when only one or two personnel are affected by an incident
- Defusing services immediately after an incident to assist crews in returning to service
- Demobilization services after a large-scale incident
- Formal Critical Incident Stress Debriefings 24 to 72 hours after an event for any emergency personnel involved in a stressful incident
- Follow-up services to assure that personnel are recovering
- Specialty debriefings to nonemergency groups on occasions when no other resources are available in a timely fashion within the community
- Support during routine discussions of an incident by emergency personnel
- Advice to command staff during large-scale events

The CISD program has been designed by an emergency person for emergency people. The CISD teams in the nation are best suited to provide support services to emergency personnel since they have been specially trained to do so.[13,14]

The authors of this book believe that Critical Incident Stress Debriefing teams are so important that an entire chapter has been developed to explain the process and procedures in greater detail. See Chapter 7 to learn more about the CISD teams and their functions.

Spouse Support Programs

The spouses of emergency personnel are in need of considerable support. They are well aware that the work their spouses perform is inherently dangerous and injuries are common. They also know that emergency workers face a higher risk of death than do people in other types of employment. These facts raise the anxiety levels of spouses. The personality features of an emergency worker cause many of them to remain silent about experiences on the job. As a result, spouses feel cut off and the stage is set for marital discord.

Both spouses and emergency personnel need improved communication skills to avoid the pitfalls of withdrawal and excessive anxiety. They frequently need education, encouragement, and sometimes counseling. When a critical incident affects an emergency worker, it also affects his or her spouse. In some instances, separate specialty debriefings have been provided to spouses after a particularly bad incident. Many organizations realize that if a worker's home life can be eased, the person may perform considerably better on the job.

Family Life Programs

Public safety agencies across the nation are beginning to realize the value of planning special educational programs, resources, and social programs designed to enhance the quality of family life for emergency services people. One useful offering would be a joint educational workshop with a title like "Coping with Stress in the Emergency Services Family" for field personnel and their spouses or other family members. Of course, these types of workshops must be led by qualified professional people to assure high quality.[15]

Counseling

Although police services have been utilizing psychologists since the mid-1960s, other emergency service agencies have only just begun to implement counseling programs for their personnel. Counseling should not be limited to job-related problems. People would benefit from a broad spectrum of counseling opportunities in a confidential environment.

Disaster Drills

Members of a Critical Incident Stress Debriefing team should be incorporated in disaster drills. They should not "mock" their intervention techniques during the drill. Role-playing their support is usually perceived as a fake, and it sets up distrust in emergency workers, who may actually need their services in the event of a disaster. What is important is that they go through the call-out procedure, be shown where to report upon arrival, and where and how to set up their support services. At most, at the conclusion of the drill, they should hand out a printed information sheet about the CISD team and its functions.

Written Policies for Mental Health Services in a Disaster

The great majority of mental health professionals are very out of place at the scene of a disaster. They are out of their natural environment and do not know what to do to be helpful. Although well meaning, the novelty of disaster work causes them to be clumsy in their interventions at the scene. In their anxiety, they may try to do too much for victims of the incident, family members of the victims, and emergency personnel. They have a belief that their mental health training has prepared them for any type of human misery. Nothing could be further from the truth. *Disaster psychology work is a specialty. It needs to be done by mental health professionals who have specialized training or it can turn into a disaster within the disaster.*[16,17]

The well-meant interventions of poorly trained mental health professionals generally come at the wrong place and time. For example, one type of mental health support, frequently called "grief counseling," is often given in the shock stage of the disaster when people are not ready for it because they are still denying the impact of the event. The "grief counseling" may do more harm than good.

At times (it is more common than we would like to admit) mental health professionals who suddenly show up at the scene are attempting to grab the limelight, be the center of media attention, and use the disaster to enhance their private practices. Without a special critical incident stress team or disaster training, they make unsubstantiated statements to the press and to the victims of the event. They usually ask the wrong questions to the wrong people at the wrong time and under the wrong circumstances. Anything which starts off with that many wrongs cannot turn out right except by accident.[18]

Effective and efficient mental health service at the scene of a disaster is no accident. It is the preplanned, organized, and trained response *team,* which has practiced the drills with the emergency response personnel, that stands the best chance of providing the right type of help at the right time.

The following guidelines are offered to organizations that are attempting to develop policies about mental health interventions at a large-scale incident or a disaster. The policies presented here are based on actual field experiences at numerous disaster sites.

- Mental health personnel should not go to a large-scale incident or a disaster unless they are either requested to go or ask permission of the command staff to go to the scene.
- Only mental health professionals who have been specially trained on CISD teams or in special disaster psychology programs should be granted *limited access* to the scene.
- Mental health professionals and their work experience should be known to the command staff. In other words, *unknown professionals do not belong at the scene.*
- Any mental health professional who does not meet the criteria above should *always* be denied access to the scene.
- Mental health professionals should report to the command center upon arrival at the scene (assuming that they have been called in) and they should request a briefing and specific instructions.
- Mental health professionals have three major functions at the scene:
    a. They provide support to *obviously distressed* personnel.
    b. They advise command staff about stress-related or psychological matters.
    c. They assist victims of the event and their families until other appropriate resources arrive.
- Mental health personnel *must stay outside the internal perimeter.*
- If under an unforeseen circumstance, they are requested to enter an internal perimeter, they must do so under direct guidance of emergency services personnel, and they should be equipped temporarily with appropriate safety equipment. They must leave the area of the internal perimeter as soon as their mission is complete.
- Mental health professionals should maintain a *very low profile.* They should not intrude into people's lives. They should limit their interventions to brief crisis-oriented support and disengage from those they are trying to help as soon as the person is stabilized and responding positively to the support or when the person's own resources have been mobilized. *They should, at all times, limit their interventions to those people who are showing obvious signs of distress.*
- Mental health personnel are serving only in an advisory capacity. They have no command authority at the scene. *Mental health professionals at an incident serve only under the authority of the commanders.*
- Any decisions regarding personnel at the scene must always have the approval of the command staff.
- Mental health professionals must never speak with media representatives at the scene without the consent of the command staff.
- Mental health professionals must have identification visible during operations at the scene.

- It is the responsibility of the mental health professional to maintain a high level of alertness and an orientation toward personal safety while engaged in field operations.
- Mental health personnel involved in a large incident would utilize their time best by setting up the demobilization center and preparing for the movement of personnel through the center (see Chapter 7 for more details on the demobilization center).

Chaplains

Chaplaincy programs are important in emergency services. However, those chosen as chaplains need to be screened carefully. Like mental health professionals, the wrong kind of help at the wrong time by the wrong people can have very negative consequences. *Chaplains would be wise to read the section on mental health services in disasters since most of what was said above has application for them as well.*

Many emergency personnel have spiritual needs which are best addressed by members of the clergy. It is a wise organization which realizes that their personnel might benefit from the support of the clergy and therefore develops a chaplaincy program within the organization. Some personnel would speak about private matters with a member of the clergy but would avoid the same kind of interaction with mental health professionals.

Periodic Stress Evaluations

It is helpful from time to time to check on how people are doing. It would be a good idea to have periodic stress evaluations of emergency personnel to make sure that they are remaining healthy. Psychological and physical aspects should be reviewed confidentiality by a mental health professional and the emergency personnel.[19]

Research

Emergency personnel are only now moving into a period of improved support services; they have frequently resisted efforts to learn more about them. To make further improvements there must be a greater openness to legitimate and well-organized studies that provide the personnel and their leadership adequate information on which to structure the development of new support programs. Researchers should provide feedback to the emergency services and assure the highest-quality research projects.

Emergency Personnel
Injury Policy

Emergency organizations would be wise to establish in advance written policies and procedures to follow when a serious line-of-duty injury occurs. Anyone can figure out that a seriously injured emergency responder must be transported to a hospital. However, many a department has been caught completely off guard when a member was seriously injured and no one knew who to notify, where and when to tell the family of the member's injury, and whether or not a family liaison was necessary. In one unfortunate case a family member was killed while rushing to a hospital to see if an injured emergency worker was all right. Perhaps a written policy stating that an officer's vehicle will be dispatched to transport the injured worker's family could save the life of a worried family member.

Line-of-Duty Death Protocol

Emergency service personnel do not like to talk about on-duty death, but it does happen. When it does, it is the most distressing situation that can befall an emergency organization. It throws the entire organization into a state of chaos which may last for many months after the incident. Policies should be written in advance and should be reviewed periodically after line-of-duty deaths in other organizations to assure that small but important details will not be overlooked. For example, it would help departments if the members had some general guidelines for removal of their dead comrade and notification of next of kin. Personnel would feel less guilty about being relieved of duty if they were given written policies which indicated that mutual-aid companies or other less involved members of the department would take over the mission once the dead member's body was removed.

Funerals

Funerals for emergency personnel are impressive as well as being sad and depressing. The ceremonies have a tremendous impact on the mourners. Most departments believe that they will never experience a line-of-duty death, so they do not plan ahead for such tragedies. A line-of-duty death will leave a department struggling to figure out what a proper emergency service funeral is all about. The severe disruption caused by not knowing what to do during such a tragic event can bring harmful criticism against an emergency organization.

Plan ahead for an official funeral. Write down details that should be attended to. Get a protocol set up in advance. It can relieve a great deal of unnecessary anxiety.

STRESS REDUCTION POLICIES

It is much easier for commanders to provide the proper support services for their personnel when *written* policies have been established in advance. Written stress management policies have a number of major advantages over verbal or "gentlemen's" agreements. They stay consistent over time and do not change every time a new commander takes the lead. They can also be applied equally to each person so that no one feels singled out for unusual treatment. Emergency personnel are more prone to go along with stress policies when they are written because they do not feel that someone is making things up as they go along. Frequently, they have had a hand in developing the policies and feel that they are therefore worthwhile pursuing. Written policies may also be utilized to train new recruits. It leaves them with far fewer questions and a lowered sense of confusion when they graduate from the academies.

Chapter 4 and this chapter present many points that can be developed into written policies. It might be advisable that commanders, or even better, a committee review the material to see what items would be most important for them to develop into written policy format. Obviously, this book cannot offer all the possible ideas that could form a well-thought-out policy. People should be creative in developing the best policies to suit their organizations and personnel.

In the following paragraphs we describe some sample policies developed by a number of public safety organizations to help keep stress at a minimum.

DIGNITARY VISITS

Dignitary visits during emergency operations are very disruptive. Vitally needed emergency personnel frequently must be diverted to provide communications, protection, transportation, and escort services to dignitaries who have chosen to drop by for a look, or worse yet, who decide that a disaster or other large-scale incident is a good opportunity to carry out some political maneuvers at the local level. A visit during the early phases of a major incident, when search, rescue, and recovery operations are under way, is irresponsible on the part of politicians and other dignitaries. The visitation practice should be totally discouraged during these phases unless dignitaries would like to assume the responsibility for disrupted emergency services which could jeopardize lives and interrupt medical care at the scene.

A policy on this issue might be written in the following manner:

> When a governmental official or other dignitary requests to come to the scene of an accident or disaster or announces an intended visit, the incident commander should inform the dignitary that a visit at that time would seriously disrupt emergency services and could jeopardize lives or interfere with medical treatment. The dignitary should be requested to delay the visit until the living victims have been removed from the scene.

> If a dignitary chooses to ignore the information provided or if an unexpected and unscheduled visit should take place, the dignitary should be requested to report to the command post and should then be assigned to a specific emergency responder who will guide the dignitary through the scene and keep him or her out of areas where there is significant risk or where delicate lifesaving operations are under way.

MEDIA

Media presence at the scene can be a major stress producer in itself. The media put emergency services personnel in the public eye. Small mistakes are frequently blown out of proportion. Interviews are demanded from distressed patients and rescuers. Evidence is disrupted. Frequently, dangers to the personnel at the scene increase because the presence of a news crew can incite certain people to riot who would normally not cause any trouble.

Many emergency personnel have the idea that they must make a statement if a camera is turned on them or if a recorder with a microphone is in front of their faces. The easiest method available to cut down on media stress is to develop a strictly enforced "media policy." Here is an example:

> While on duty at an incident, no emergency services person shall allow himself or herself to be interviewed or make any statement about the incident or the operations to any media representative(s) without the consent of the incident commander. Failure to comply with this directive will result in disciplinary action.

> If members of the media are requesting information from any emergency services person, that person will politely direct the media representative to the designated public information officer and decline any further requests to pro-

vide information about the incident or the operations. Preincident agreements and guidelines with local media should be made to reduce problems.

SUMMARY

The emphasis in this chapter was on providing administrators and commanders with some insights into a broad spectrum of stress reduction strategies which could easily be developed and implemented by the emergency organizations. It was suggested that administrators and command staff remain open to learning new, improved management tactics, including interactive leadership. It was also suggested that some effort be put into the development of employee assistance programs, family life programs, chaplaincy programs, and preplanned mental health support strategies.

Chapter 6 will point out a variety of important stress reduction techniques that should be employed over one's entire life span. The responsibility for personal stress reduction falls squarely on the heads of the individuals, although the organization can be supportive, as pointed out in this chapter.

REFERENCES

1. Sundberg, N. D. (1977). *Assessment of Persons*. Englewood Cliffs, NJ: Prentice-Hall.
2. Everly, G. S., and Sobelman, S. A. (1987). *Assessment of Human Stress Response*. New York: AMS Press.
3. Millon, T., and Everly, G. (1985). *Personality and Its Disorders*. New York: Wiley.
4. Aiken, L. R. (1985). *Psychological Testing and Assessment*. Boston: Allyn and Bacon.
5. Mitchell, J. T. (1981). *Emergency Response to Crisis*. Bowie, MD: R. J. Brady Co.
6. Mitchell, J. T. (1988). The impact of stress on emergency service personnel: Policy issues in emergency response. In L. K. Comfort, Ed., *Managing Disasters*. Durham, NC: Duke University Press.
7. Steinmetz, J., et al. (1980). *Managing Stress before It Manages You*. Palo Alto, CA: Bull Publishing Co.
8. McConnell, E. A. (1982). *Burnout in the Nursing Profession: Coping Strategies, Causes and Costs*. St. Louis: C. V. Mosby.
9. Cooper, C. L. (1981). *Executive Families under Stress: How Male and Female Managers Can Keep Their Pressures Out of Their Homes*. Englewood Cliffs, NJ: Prentice-Hall.

10. Monk, T. H., and Folkard, S. (1983). Circadian rhythms and shiftwork. In R. Hockey (Ed.), *Stress and Fatigue in Human Performance.* New York: Wiley.

11. Culligan, M. J., and Sedlacek, K. (1980). *How to Avoid Stress before It Kills You.* New York: Gramercy Publishing Co.

12. Mitchell, J. T. (1986). Teaming up against critical stress. *Chief Fire Executive, 1*(1): 24; 36; 84.

13. Mitchell, J. T. (1983). When disaster strikes: The critical incident stress debriefing process. *Journal of Emergency Medical Services, 8*(1): 36–39.

14. Mitchell, J. T. (1985). Healing the helper. In B. Greene (Ed.), *Role Stressors and Supports for Emergency Workers.* Washington, DC: Center for Mental Health Studies of Emergencies, U.S. Department of Health and Human Services.

15. Harris, V. (1988). Coping with stress in the emergency services family. Presented Apr. 6, 1988, for the Howard County, Maryland, Fire Department.

16. Raphael, B. (1986). *When Disaster Strikes: How Individuals and Communities Cope with Catastrophe.* New York: Basic Books.

17. Comfort, L. K. (Ed.). (1988). *Managing Disaster: Strategies and Rating Perspectives.* Durham, NC: Duke University Press.

18. Bradford, G., et al. (1988). Dealing with bystanders. *Emergency Medical Services, The Journal of Emergency Care and Transportation, 17*(1): 17, 18; 20–23; 26.

19. Matteson, M. T., and Ivancevich, J. (1982). *Managing Job Stress and Health.* New York: Free Press.

6

LIFELONG STRESS MANAGEMENT STRATEGIES

Service organizations have a vested interest in maintaining healthy responders. Their interventions for volunteers or career employees (see Chapter 5) are designed to minimize absenteeism, personal disruption, and low productivity while maximizing quality of work life, competency, and personal satisfaction. *Organizational interventions are not sufficient to resolve the major sources of stress for emergency workers. To attack these potentially destructive influences successfully, emergency responders must accept primary responsibility for themselves.*[1]

DIET

The United States is a country of the fat obsessed with the lean. Unfortunately, the same issue exists within the ranks of emergency responders. The problems associated with improper diet can, however, have more devastating consequences for emergency service providers than for the general public. If they are eating foods that cause their health to deteriorate, or foods that increase their stress, they, and the public they serve, will be subject to increased dangers from their compromised performance, stamina, and lowered ability to tolerate stress.

Proper diet is a major concern in any comprehensive stress management program. A proper diet ensures that the nutritional resources for growth, healing, energy, and health are readily available, while limiting harmful substances such as refined sugars, caffeine, fats (cholesterol/triglycerides), and excessive salt, which almost always intensify stress.[2]

101

Stress-Producing Foods

Some foods contain substances capable of directly stimulating the stress response in the body. If a person eats foods containing these substances (called *sympathomimetic agents* because they stimulate the sympathetic nervous system), their bodies respond as if they were experiencing some significant stressor in the environment.[3,4]

Caffeine

The most common sympathomimetic or stress-producing substance that people consume is caffeine. In the presence of caffeine, heart rate changes, blood pressure elevates, and there is an increased need for oxygen. In addition, caffeine directly stimulates cardiac muscle tissue and the central nervous system. Headaches, diarrhea, anxiety, cardiac arrhythmias, nervousness, irritability, and sleeplessness may also result when caffeine is present in the body. Any amount of caffeine greater than 250 milligrams per day is considered excessive and almost always causes negative effects. Some people will react to caffeine at considerably smaller doses. It should be noted that the average coffee drinker consumes two or more six-ounce cups of coffee per day. Each cup contains approximately 110 milligrams of caffeine. This amount of caffeine is added to the amounts obtained from other sources of caffeine in the diet, such as chocolate, tea, some over-the-counter medications, and cola beverages. The total caffeine intake for many people may easily exceed the 250 milligrams, which is considered excessive. *For less stress, lighten up on the caffeine intake.*[1-4]

Other Foods Associated
with Increased Stress

A careless approach to nutrition is one of the principal contributors to stress in emergency personnel. Emergency personnel would never even consider deliberately putting the wrong type of lubricants or fuels in the equipment they use or the vehicles they drive. Yet they do not think twice when filling themselves full of the wrong kinds of fuel for their bodies and the type of work they are required to perform. There are other foods that have either direct or indirect association with stress, whose use should be limited in one's diet. Excessive amounts of these substances in a person's diet may limit an emergency responder from performing at his or her peak.

Alcohol

At no time should alcohol be consumed while on duty. It has direct negative effects on one's performance, behavior, judgment, and physical coordination. On-duty use of alcohol is always a dangerous activity which may lead to physical, emotional, and legal consequences.

Additionally, alcohol leaves people more vulnerable to stress reactions. It is a toxic substance that is metabolized by the liver. The metabolic process uses up vitamins B and C. Vitamins B and C are essential in the production of proteins, which, in turn, are the building blocks of antibodies and white blood cells. Antibodies and white blood cells are one of the primary defense systems of the body. Depletion of vitamins B and C leave the body more vulnerable to stress and disease. Alcohol also directly suppresses protein synthesis in the body and thus leaves it more vulnerable to the harmful effects of stress.[5-7]

To avoid making a bad situation worse, people should not drink when they are stressed, anxious, depressed, and/or angry. They should also not drink alcohol out of habit. If a person wants to drink, he or she should drink slowly, in moderation, and in the context of a social interaction that they would enjoy even if they were not drinking.

If emergency workers are finding that they have to drink alcohol to manage the stress of the emergency services job, they are probably in emotional pain and undoubtedly need professional support. Use of alcohol, or any drug substance for that matter, to assist in coping with a job is akin to self-medication for pain. It is a bad choice and should be rethought quickly. Persons who cannot stop drinking on their own need professional help (which is readily available in the majority of communities in the nation).[2]

Sugar

Sugar is a major ingredient in the American diet. Its consumption is surpassed only by those of flour and meat. It contributes directly to obesity and dental problems. There may also be a link between sugar and diabetes and heart disease. To metabolize sugar in the body B-complex vitamins must be available. If a person consumes too much sugar, B-complex vitamins will be depleted in the body. The nervous and endocrine systems suffer most from depletion of B-complex vitamins. These systems are, of course, vital in the stress response. But the problems with sugar do not end there. Sugar is associated with an increased vulnerability to stress through a process called the "hypoglycemia phenomenon."[2,8,9]

Hypoglycemia occurs when the level of glucose (sugar in the blood) gets too low. It is characterized by a variety of symptoms, but especially anxiety, headaches, dizziness, trembling, and increased cardiac activity. People can develop a hypoglycemic condition either by skipping meals or by eating excessive sugar. *When hypoglycemia develops, routine stimuli that would normally not bother a person may become extremely stressful.* A hypoglycemic person becomes extremely irritable and impatient and has a significantly lowered tolerance for stress. Hungry people are notoriously irritable.

There are two types of hypoglycemia. The first, "functional hypoglycemia," originates when people skip meals. It can be made worse by high-sugar-content snack food. The second type of hypoglycemia, "reactive hypoglycemia," occurs when people consume high levels of sugar in a short period. It seems paradoxical that a high volume of sugar could actually cause a condition of low blood sugar, but that is exactly what happens.

The body reacts to a high-sugar condition (hypoglycemia) in the following manner. As high levels of sugar enter the bloodstream, insulin is released by the pancreas. The insulin signals the body's tissues to allow the blood sugar to enter all the tissues of the body. Blood sugar is not reserved for the central nervous system, which depends heavily on it for its function. Once the blood sugar (glucose) enters the body's tissues, its level in the bloodstream decreases dramatically and a hypoglycemic condition results.

When the intake of sugar is extremely high, the symptoms of hypoglycemia may manifest themselves in a brief period. They may also be quite serious and produce nausea, staggering, slurred speech, and fainting. All of these signs have been noted at incidents where emergency personnel have eaten lots of sugary snack foods in a brief period. The best way to avoid the problems associated with hypoglycemia is to eat regularly scheduled, well-balanced meals that contain a minimum of sugar and processed foods (which usually contain a great deal of hidden sugar).[2,4]

Salt

Sodium chloride (salt) is important in the regulation of the body's water balance. But too much of it is extremely hazardous to human health. In the presence of high levels of salt, fluid tends to build up in the body and to set the stage for high blood pressure. High blood pressure substantially increases the risk of stroke and heart attack. Additionally, excessive fluid retention in the body tends to increase fluid-caused pressure in the central nervous system (brain and spinal cord). This leads to an increase of nervous tension and feelings of irritability. *Increased salt leads to an increased potential for increased stress.* Cutting salt intake helps to maintain health.[1,2]

Processed Flour

The processed flour that is the basis of many breads, pastries, gravy, and other foods has been implicated as a vitamin robber. The various processing procedures remove most of the essential nutrients in the grains. The nutrients destroyed include the B-complex vitamins, vitamin E, and minerals such as calcium, phosphorus, potassium, and magnesium.

White bread is the most serious robber of the essential nutrients described above. Not only is it made of nutrient-poor processed flour, but it also contains a great deal of salt and sugar. White bread is a "loser" on a number of counts. *Emergency personnel would be well advised to switch to whole-grain breads if they would like to eat a healthier diet.*[2,10]

Cholesterol

Diets with large volumes of cholesterol contribute to deteriorated health and potentially higher levels of stress. Cholesterol comes from such foods as eggs, cheese, shrimp, crab, and any food substance that is high in animal fat. Americans eat so many foods containing high levels of cholesterol that it is estimated that our serum cholesterol levels are as much as 100 to 200 percent higher than those of peoples in many other parts of the world. High levels of cholesterol in the blood are associated with considerably increased potential for heart disease.

Cholesterol is deposited on the wall of the arteries and causes them to narrow and limit blood flow to the organs of the body. There are two types of cholesterol:

1. Low-density lipoproteins
2. High-density lipoproteins

Low-density lipoproteins are found in the deposits that clog arteries. High-density lipoproteins have the ability to dissolve low-density lipoproteins. So a healthy person aims at a lower ratio of low-density cholesterol to higher-density cholesterol. Some evidence now exists that the overall level of low-density lipoproteins can be lowered with a careful diet. But even more important in lowering low-density cholesterol is an increase in physical exercise.[2,11]

Vitamins Are Important in Stress Control

During periods of stress high levels of vitamin C and the B-complex vitamins [thiamine (B_1), riboflavin (B_2), niacin, pantothenic acid (B_5), pyridoxine hydrochloride (B_6), and choline] are essential if the nervous and endocrine systems are to continue to function properly. These vitamins are not only essential to create the appropriate stress response in the body, but also become victims of excessive stress and become depleted. Deficiencies of these vitamins will lead to a decreased ability by the body to respond properly to stress. Lowered or depleted levels of vitamins B_1, B_5, and B_6 may cause heightened emotional responses such as intensified anxiety reactions, depression, insomnia, and cardiovascular weakness. Vitamin deficiencies in B_2 and niacin may cause stomach irritability and general weakness of the muscles. These signs of physical distress are not uncommon during emergencies. *The end result of vitamin deficiency is a lowered tolerance for stress.*

Vitamin supplements are recommended to lower the chances of vitamin depletion in stressed people and to better prepare the body to manage stress when it occurs. Vitamin C and the B-complex vitamins are the most important. Some companies manufacture a "stress" vitamin supplement which is high in the vitamins typically depleted by stress reactions. *However, vitamins should be a supplement and not a substitute for good nutrition.*

Dietary Guidelines

The following guidelines will be helpful to anyone who is trying to improve his or her nutrition.[2,3,12] They are particularly helpful for emergency personnel.

1. Avoid sugar, salt, white breads, alcohol, and caffeine as much as possible.
2. Increase the consumption of complex carbohydrates, such as whole grain breads, granola, bran, so that the total calories from carbohydrates in the diet is closer to 48 percent than its current average of 28 percent.
3. Dramatically reduce the intake of fatty foods. Avoid or reduce consumption of fried foods, nuts, fatty meats, chips, and other foods high in fat.
4. Watch especially the intake of foods that are known to be loaded with cholesterol, such as eggs, cheese, shrimp, crab, and butter. (The dietary needs of children and elderly may vary and exceptions may need to be made.)
5. Utilize polyunsaturated and monosaturated fats instead of saturated fats.
6. Aim at a 50 percent reduction of refined sugars.
7. Reduce salt intake by 15 to 70 percent, depending on current consumption.
8. Try to eat only as many calories as are expended in a day.
9. If overweight, decrease food intake and increase exercise.
10. Increase the consumption of fruits and vegetables and whole grains.
11. Except for young children, substitute low fat and nonfat milk for whole milk. Also use low-fat dairy products.
12. Consume more fish and poultry.
13. Become a label reader and watch out for foods that have a high hidden salt or sugar content.
14. Increase exercise as needed to assist with weight control and to maintain a high level of physical fitness.

15. Use multivitamin supplements, but do not over do it.
16. Avoid crash diets.
17. Check with your physician before dieting.
18. Once you lose weight you have to be careful not to revert to poor eating habits. It will be necessary to maintain proper nutrition and proper exercise to keep the weight off.

EXERCISE

Emergency people have jobs that are among the most stressful in the world. The demands of emergency response require the utmost in psychological as well as physical stamina. Sadly, many emergency personnel have ignored their own good health and have eaten badly and avoided any regular exercise. They have allowed themselves to grow soft in mind and body. When called upon to protect others, save a life, or fight a fire, they frequently are not up to the task. They huff and puff throughout the crisis event and everyone hopes they will make it through. A review of the statistics regarding the causes of death of emergency personnel can be quite shocking. Aside from police officers, who usually die as a result of violence, the majority of emergency personnel who die in the line of duty die as a result of cardiac arrest, which is secondary to stress-related causes. In fact, it is estimated that approximately 50 percent of the premature deaths in the United States result from a combination of two factors: smoking and physical inactivity. Many emergency service deaths, including those of police officers, could be prevented if the responders were more physically fit. It is very sad to lose so many good personnel through their neglect of self.

Many people would like to skip this section. They think that physical exercise is much too much to ask of them. They do not realize that it is not as difficult as they might imagine. Just walking a mile a day can substantially reduce the risk of dying prematurely. So read on; there may be a few other pointers here from which you can benefit.

Numerous studies have pointed to significant benefits of regular physical exercise. Some of the key benefits are:

- Increased muscular strength and stamina
- Enhanced heart and lung capacity
- Decreased heart rate and blood pressure
- Replacement of fat with muscle
- Improved self-esteem

- Increased red blood cells and oxygen profusion to the tissues
- Improved sleep
- Improved weight control
- Lowered cholesterol levels
- Reduced use of alcohol and tobacco
- Reduced severity of injury should an injury occur
- Reduced probability of injury during emergency operations

The entire stress response has been designed for physical activity. The most effective means of dealing with stress is to utilize physical action. A person who recognizes this fact and then utilizes physical activity has the advantage of quickly calming or channeling the flood of chemicals in the body which are associated with the stress response and which are frequently caustic to the tissues of the body. (See Chapter 1 for more details on the physiological response to stress.)

Research indicates that people who utilize physical exertion exercise report very low or no tension after strenuous exercise. Anxiety has also been lowered by exercise. People who exercise regularly generally have more stable emotional states; they feel less depressed and less angry.[1,2,13]

Aerobic Exercise

The aim of physical exercise should be to reach and maintain an aerobic state for twenty minutes. Aerobic activity is any activity in which large volumes of oxygen are used by the body. Under conditions of certain consistent strenuous activities the body takes in great amounts of oxygen. The oxygen profusion to the tissues of the body improves their function and eliminates chemicals that have accumulated during periods of physical inactivity and mental stress.

Aerobic exercise has the following characteristics:

- Exercise is performed at least three times a week.
- Exercise should increase the heart rate to a minimum of 70 percent of maximum.
- Exercise should be maintained for twenty minutes.

More will be said on aerobic exercise in the section to follow.

Aerobic Exercise
and Heart Rate

It can be very dangerous for people to simply begin exercising vigorously when they have not been on a regular exercise program. It is especially dangerous if they are over 35 years old and have been leading a rather sedentary life-style. *The very first step a person should take before beginning a regular exercise program is to get a checkup by a physician.*

Over time the exercise program gradually increases in intensity. The aim is to build up to a minimum of 70 percent of one's maximum heart rate, which is the minimum level of aerobic exercise that will have a training effect. Then a person gradually increases the aerobic exercise until 85 percent of maximum cardiac activity is attained. The 85 percent of maximum cardiac rate is the most recommended level of aerobic exercise. For some people who are extremely fit, a 95 percent level may be obtained. However, *no one should attempt to reach 95 percent maximum of cardiac rate without a physician's approval.*[2,15] Figure 6–1 should be helpful in determining the cardiac rate appropriate for one's age and level of physical fitness.

Types of Exercise

Walking   This is a very good beginning exercise. Pick a good time of the day and stick to it. Walk on a regular basis. A mile or two a day is a good goal. Some people have benefitted from as little as a quarter of a mile a day.

Running   Check with your physician before training as a runner. Running is well known for its aerobic benefits. When worked at consistently, it has many positive benefits. But there are some hazards to running and people need to receive the proper medical advice before getting into it.

Swimming   More muscle groups are involved in swimming than in running. It is at least as beneficial as running as an aerobic exercise. It is not as convenient as running because it depends on having a facility available year round.

Calisthenics and Weight Training   These are excellent for developing muscle tone, cardiac output, and general physical stamina. Excellent stress dissipaters.

FIGURE 6–1   Exercise and Heart Rate

For any physical activity to produce positive cardiovascular effects, it must increase your heart rate. What the proper heart rate is depends on such factors as sex, age, and physical conditions. Use the chart below to determine what your target rate should be.

100% is your maximum possible heart rate.

95% is a rate you should reach *only* if you are in a top level of fitness for your age.

85% is the generally recommended level to reach during physical activity.

70% is the minimum level that must be reached for any training effect to occur.

Age	100%		95%		85%		70%	
	Male	Female	Male	Female	Male	Female	Male	Female
20	195	205	186	195	165	174	137	144
25	190	200	181	190	162	170	133	140
30	185	195	176	185	158	166	130	137
35	180	190	171	180	154	162	126	133
40	175	185	166	175	149	157	123	130
45	170	180	161	170	145	153	119	126
50	165	175	156	165	141	148	116	123
55	160	170	151	160	137	145	112	119
60	155	165	146	155	132	140	109	116
65	150	160	141	150	128	136	105	112

Reprinted with permission of The Free Press, a Division of Macmillan, Inc. from *Managing Job Stress and Health: The Intelligent Person's Guide* by Michael T. Matteson and John M. Ivancevich. Copyright © 1982 by The Free Press.

Tennis, Golf, Handball   If you walk when playing golf, you have moderate physical exercise. Tennis and handball (doubles) are also moderate in their ability to exercise the body. Tennis and handball (singles) are in the vigorous category and therefore provide good physical activity. The problem with these sports is that they are competitive and a stress-prone individual may lose the goal of enjoyment and attend only to the goal of winning. If that is the case, more stress may be generated by the sports than is reduced by them. Do not choose these types of activities if you are already stress prone.

Other Good Exercises   Cross-country skiing, bicycling, canoeing, hiking, downhill skiing, martial arts, mountain climbing, gardening and household chores, and general activities all provide exercise. *The important thing is to be active and to enjoy what you are doing.*

General Guidelines for Physical Exercise
- Get a physical examination first.
- Follow the physician's advice.
- Start very slowly and build up gradually.
- Train. Do not strain.
- Rest properly. Get plenty of sleep.
- If it is causing pain, stop and get checked.
- Always warm up—include muscle stretching.
- Buy the right shoes and other equipment.
- Be regular (twenty minutes three times a week).
- Have fun or it is not worth doing.[1,2,4,14,15]

STOP SMOKING

The use of tobacco products is directly and indirectly associated with increased stress. Tobacco contains nicotine. Like caffeine, nicotine has direct effects on the sympathetic nervous system. Nicotine is classified as one of the sympathomimetic chemicals and can cause the same negative reactions that people would get from caffeine (see the section on caffeine earlier in this chapter). Nicotine stimulates the adrenal glands and they release hormones that produce the stress response in the body. The heart rate increases, blood pressure rises, fatty acids pour into the bloodstream, and blood glucose increases. Nicotine also depletes vitamins C and E. As pointed out earlier, depletion of these vitamins causes the body to be less ready to cope with stress.

Not only is the smoker in danger, but those who breathe the smoke are also in danger. Nicotine enters the body through smoke. One's spouse, children, friends, and coworkers are exposed to a chemical that directly increases their stress and reduces the ability of their bodies to fight off disease.

Volumes of evidence exist which point out clearly that smoking is the greatest cause of preventable death in the United States today. It is directly associated with lung cancer and other respiratory diseases. It is also associated with increased coronary disease. *Continued smoking in light of this mounting evidence is irresponsible and self-destructive.* Unfortunately, many innocent people, including children, must suffer the consequences of the smoker's self-destruction. Remember the saying: "When mother or father smokes, baby chokes."

Emergency workers who smoke are making themselves far more vulnerable to serious stress problems. It is difficult to believe they would want to do that since they may become less capable of performing their jobs when more highly stressed.

Here is a basic rule regarding smoking as a direct enhancer of the stress response. *If you have never smoked—do not start. If you are a smoker—quit now.* Your families and friends will be grateful.

Chewing Tobacco

Chewing tobacco is not a good substitute for smoking. It has similar health risks as smoking. There is also increased risks for contagious disease when the product is spit.

EXHILARATION

Exhilaration is the process of turning the negative aspects of the stress reaction around and making them positive. It is accomplished when people begin to feel that they are in charge of their situation and decide not to allow stress to beat them. Exhilaration can be achieved by a combination of two things. The first is to follow the guidelines outlined thus far in this chapter which relate to proper diet, exercise, and the cessation of smoking. Those stress reduction strategies will do much to help the emergency person to have a less tense environment and more positive view of the world. As their confidence builds and their self-esteem rises, they can then move into the second activity which helps to bring them into a state of exhilaration.[16]

The second item which must be accomplished to generate exhilaration is the adjustment of one's mental attitude. People have to start seeing stress as a challenge to be overcome, not as something awful that controls their life. Exhilaration comes about when people finally believe that they are in control and have the potential to overcome and beat stress. Many of the strategies in the remainder of this chapter and the chapters to follow will help emergency personnel to feel more in control of their own destiny.

TAPPING INTERNAL RESOURCES

Human beings have a great deal more power inside themselves than they realize. If they could tap into their internal resources, they would be able to accomplish great things and reduce their stress reactions substantially. Human beings can think, categorize, remember, mentally visualize a situation, see the humor in something, and can decide which things are worth getting upset about and which things are not. They can also use their thinking processes when their emotions are out of line and need to be brought under control.

Human beings have a conscience and they would be wise to listen to themselves and not do things which they find inherently uncomfortable. Much stress is produced by people who have developed guilt because they have *deliberately* done things which they felt at the time they should not do and which they later regretted. (Guilt related to a *mistake* is usually an unnecessary distortion of the facts and can be alleviated by an objective review of the true facts related to a situation.)

To reduce stress, people need to use their thinking process for reason, judgment, and prudence; they need to use their humor; they should not avoid their conscience but should use it well. Emergency people could help themselves a great deal if they decided which battles were really worth fighting. Many times they become embroiled in controversies at work that are not solvable and are worthless to pursue. They use their limited resources to fight unwinnable battles. The result is intensified cumulative stress reactions (see Chapters 2 and 3) and a limited ability to deal with acute stress under field conditions. Sometimes they get so hung up over small, worthless battles that they are unable to perform properly at the scene of an incident. A few may hesitate to follow the legitimate commands of an officer because they are involved in a conflict back at the station.[17]

Tap into inner strengths to reduce stress. The overall results may be amazing to those who try them out. Some strategies to improve one's use of inner resources are described in the paragraphs that follow.

Relaxation

Relaxation is not the same thing as rest. Relaxation is a more purposeful quieting of the mind and the body than simply sitting down and resting or sleeping. Relaxation allows a recovery from stress which is more effective than rest alone. Relaxation stimulates the production of chemicals in the body which have the effect of neutralizing the stress chemicals described in Chapter 1. Relaxation can be achieved by several methods:[18]

- Deep breathing
- Progressive muscle relaxation
- Biofeedback
- Visual imagery
- Hypnosis
- Meditation

Some of the techniques that have been found to be most useful to emergency personnel are described in some detail below. That does not mean that the other techniques are not useful—they are. But they are either less immediately effective for emergency personnel or they are not usually utilized by emergency personnel because some of the techniques do not fit the general personality characteristics of most emergency personnel. If you are practicing some of the techniques not described in detail in the following paragraphs, keep up the good work. If you would like to begin using other techniques, not mentioned here refer to some of the books and articles in the references at the end of the chapter.

Deep Breathing

Taking in a deep breath and then blowing it out forcefully seems to be a natural stress control technique. With a little training the natural process of deep breathing when a person is under stress can be improved and made more effective. Deep breathing has been taught to police officers and they have used it with considerable success under both emergency and nonemergency conditions.[19] There are basically three levels of breathing:

- Very deep breathing
- Deep breathing
- Normal breathing

The objective of breathing exercises is to inhale breaths through the nose and exhale them through the mouth, with the lips pursed to provide some resistance. Instead of breathing as one normally would, efforts are made to hold each breath for a brief period before exhaling it somewhat forcefully.

Starting with the deepest breaths first, the person inhales the very deepest possible breath through the nose, holds the breath for five seconds, and then exhales through the mouth with the lips pursed. Then they relax their body as much as possible and breathe normally for five to eight seconds. Then another breath is taken in, held, and finally released in the same manner. Very deep breathing is repeated three times with a brief pause between each breath.

Next, the person goes into deep breathing. The breaths are smaller in volume than the very deep breaths described above. They are roughly one-half the volume of the very deep breaths. They are inhaled in the same manner as the very deep breaths, that is, through the nose. However, they are held a bit longer—usually eight to ten seconds—before they are forcefully exhaled through the pursed lips. Like the very deep breaths, deep breaths are repeated three times.

The last stage in the breathing relaxation process is to breathe in normal-sized breaths. These breaths are full-sized normal breaths, not the exaggerated deep breaths of the deep and very deep processes in the preceding paragraphs. Again they are brought in through the nose, held, and then exhaled forcefully through the mouth with the same kind of resistance as described above. The only thing which is different is that the normal-sized breaths are held longer—approximately ten to fifteen seconds for normal-sized breaths. Like the two sets of breathing exercises described above, the normal breaths are repeated three times.

Deep breathing has one main advantage for emergency personnel. It may be practiced before, during, or after an incident. The eyes do not have to be closed nor does the person have to be lying down. The entire process can be shortened if circumstances warrant it. For example, only the very deep breaths might be needed, or one breath from each of the three styles could be utilized. With enough practice, some people are able to get some calming effect with only one very deep breath.[18-20]

Progressive Muscle Relaxation

Tension and relaxation cannot exist in the same muscles at the same time. That principle underlies the use of progressive muscle relaxation as a stress reduction strategy. Progressive muscle relaxation exercises call for an exaggerated tensing of a particular muscle group. The exaggerated tension in a muscle group signals the brain that the muscles are too tight. The brain then begins a process by which "relaxation" chemicals enter the bloodstream and neutralize or lessen the stress reaction. What happens in progressive muscle relaxation is that the exaggerated tightening of the muscles "fools" the brain into initiating the relaxation response instead of the stress response.[21]

To utilize progressive muscle relaxation procedures, the following steps should be taken. Begin at the lower extremities, tensing the muscles of the feet and ankles first. Then move to the muscle groups that are located in the calves of the legs, then the thighs, buttocks, and abdomen. Finally, the muscle groups in the lower back, chest, and upper back are worked before moving into the arms, neck, and head and facial muscles. The basic idea is to tighten each successive muscle group in an exaggerated fashion but without producing pain. The muscle tension is held for five seconds before being released. Each muscle group is flexed or extended two times with a brief five-second pause between each exercise. Once muscle groups are relaxed, the effects usually last for a while before the tension returns. The more a person practices muscle relaxation, the longer the effects last.

The entire progressive muscle relaxation process, and many other stress reduction strategies, are detailed in a book by Daniel Girdano and George Everly entitled *Controlling Stress and Tension,* 2nd edition (Englewood Cliffs, NJ: Prentice-Hall, 1986). It is strongly recommended for people who want to know how to do the procedure properly. Describing the entire process here would make this book too lengthy. We have outlined the process here simply to indicate that it is a stress reduction strategy which has particular usefulness for emergency people.

Biofeedback and Hypnosis

Biofeedback and hypnosis are both very effective in cutting down on stress reactions. They are quite effective with emergency personnel. The only drawback to using them is that they require some training and, in the case of biofeedback, some equipment in their early stages. They are highly recommended stress reduction techniques, but people should be careful to choose well-qualified coaches to get them properly trained and working on their own.[22,23]

Visual Imagery
and Meditation

Visual imagery and meditation are also very useful techniques for achieving stress reduction. However, because they require some training, people wishing to use them need both dedication and patience. Many emergency people do not have the type of personality that is compatible with sitting still long enough to learn how to do visual imagery and meditation and to practice it regularly once they learn it.

Most relaxation quieting and visual imagery techniques require the following:

- A quiet environment free of distractions
- A passive attitude that allows the mind and body to stay quiet
- A comfortable position

• A mental device such as a word that is repeated to help the person avoid distractions

People who meditate are urged to keep their minds free of thoughts and to keep their bodies still and quiet. Busy emergency personnel could be very refreshed by eliminating the feeling that they have to be up and doing something at every moment of every day.

Visual imagery is a technique by which people imagine themselves doing something they enjoy very much in a relaxed and quiet place. Imagining calm, relaxed states often helps a person to feel calm and relaxed. Some people might like to try meditation and/or visual imagery but are not sure they could do it. Figure 6-2 should be helpful to them in making a decision as to whether meditation or guided imagery is a good technique for them to follow.[2,24]

FIGURE 6-2 Do You Have Good Imagery Skills?

Some people are better than others at creating clear mental images. Test yourself by responding to the following items. Read an item and then try to imagine that item as clearly as you can. Rate your image a *1* if it is unclear; a *2* if it is fairly clear; a *3* if it is very clear.

1. Imagine the face of a close friend or relative.
2. Picture a baked turkey ready for carving.
3. Feel the warmth of a hot shower.
4. Picture the house in which you grew up.
5. Taste a glass of cool lemonade.
6. Imagine a field of wildflowers blowing in the breeze.
7. Smell the aroma of spaghetti sauce cooking.
8. Picture yourself driving a race car at Indianapolis.
9. Feel your bare feet walking along a sandy beach.
10. Imagine the sound of a dog barking.

Scoring: 25 or more	You have well-developed powers of imagery.
13 to 24	You could stand some practice.
12 or less	Practice won't help — you need special training.

Reprinted with permission of The Free Press, a Division of Macmillan, Inc. from *Managing Job Stress and Health: The Intelligent Person's Guide* by Michael T. Matteson and John M. Ivancevich. Copyright © 1982 by The Free Press.

Spirituality

Human spirituality is a particularly individual thing. People have their own beliefs and generally resent attempts from others to influence those beliefs. No attempt is made here to question or to influence anyone, one way or the other, about their beliefs. What is noted is the fact that spirituality or a personal beliefs system can be very effective for some people as a method of stress reduction.

People who have a belief in an afterlife, and those who believe that there is a benign and caring force or power or being or God, who is concerned about the needs, activities, and feelings of human beings, tend to be able to cope well with high degrees of stress for longer periods. It is as if having a belief in a power beyond themselves gives them extra strength and endurance. For many, their personal spirituality gives special meaning to their lives. It provides explanations and answers for them which others may not enjoy. Stress may be viewed from a new perspective.

Emergency personnel are encouraged to pursue their own spiritual base. Prayer, meditation, contemplation, religious ceremony, and a personal belief system are extremely important for a person's health. People are not made up simply of their physical bodies and their thoughts and emotions. They are whole only when their spiritual beliefs are incorporated into the other aspects of their being. Stress is lowered when people feel in harmony and balance in all aspects of their life. We hope that the spiritual side will not be ignored, since it may offer much to a person's health.

LIFE BEYOND THE JOB

Apart from critical incidents that suddenly overwhelm a person's ability to cope with an intensely stressful situation, most of the stress encountered by emergency personnel arises from a life out of balance. For some, their emergency work has become the all-important thing in life. Its importance far surpasses the importance of the family and of other pursuits. Some emergency workers experience not only a career job in emergency services, but also have other emergency-oriented activities. Some join volunteer emergency units to have a place to spend their time after they have finished their shifts on their regular job. Still others need to be in several emergency fields simultaneously. They may be career police officers and part-time or volunteer firefighter and ambulance personnel or dispatchers.

Although they are particularly well suited by personality to perform these tasks, they may actually set themselves up for more debilitating stress reactions simply by the amount of exposure they have to distressing calls. They may be trying to live eighty years of life in only 20 years. Every other aspect of their life begins to suffer from excessive exposure to the emergency fields. Families, friendships, hobbies, household maintenance, sports, and even their health may become unimportant and forgotten.

A person who does not have a life beyond the job has a life out of balance. When they are pained by their constant exposure to emergency sit uations, they find they have no one to whom to turn. They end up alone, without friends or family to assist them, and they may seek relief in alcohol or other drugs of abuse. They realize too late that had they poured even half as much energy into their marriages and friendships, they would not now be alone.

It would be in the best interests of emergency personnel if they could find a way to modify their drive for exposure to emergency events. People who survive in emergency services are those who have learned to pace them-selves throughout their life and over the entire span of their careers. They realize that there is a life beyond the job and that that life offers them sup-port, security, safety, nourishment, a replenishing of their energy, peace, and fun.

LIMITED SELF-DISCLOSURE

Emergency workers would be wise to discuss their reactions, feelings, and thoughts following an emergency situation that has been particularly dis-tressing. Discussion of the event may not be their normal style. However, they have much to gain if they can open up a little to fellow team members, family members, and trusted friends. The ability to talk about a bad call frequently puts things in perspective. Emergency personnel usually feel less unique in their reactions once they are able to talk about them. They begin to see that others who were at the scene have similar reactions. Their re-actions appear more normal when they realize that they are not alone in having them.

Early discussions of the critical incident in either an initial discussion or a small-group defusing are encouraged. Those discussions may be suf-ficient to clear up a great deal of the distress associated with a call before stress reactions become set and more difficult to deal with (see Chapter 7).

Sometimes the initial discussion of an event leads into a defusing ses-sion in which a specially trained peer support person or mental health profes-sional may be brought in to lead a brief crew discussion. The intent of such a discussion is to assist the crew in bringing out some of the more distressing elements of a call. But, more important, the leader of the defusing presents suggestions that can be utilized by the crew members to reduce their reactions to the situation.

In some cases, the critical incident is more powerful and the stress reactions stirred up by the event may need to be addressed in a more formalized structured approach called a Critical Incident Stress Debriefing (CISD; see Chapter 7 for a more detailed description of the process). The CISD takes place after twenty-four hours, unlike the initial discussion or the defusing session, which occurs within a few hours of the incident. The CISD is led by a team of specially trained mental health professionals and peer support personnel. It helps to lessen the impact of the event and it accelerates the recovery of the personnel. It is a good opportunity for personnel to ventilate their feelings and to obtain some important information from knowledgeable people which can be immediately helpful to them in controlling and reducing their stress reactions.

In initial discussions, defusings, and debriefings (see Chapter 7 for more information) the emphasis is on limited self-disclosure. This means that emergency personnel talk about their own experiences, emotions, and thoughts regarding the incident they just experienced. Although it is not an easy thing for emergency personnel to do, most who have been able to talk about a critical incident usually realize that they are experiencing a strong feeling of relief once the unspeakable has been said. The hardest part is getting past the fear that others will view them as weak, strange, mentally ill (crazy), incompetent, or different as a result of their reaction to a particular event.

That last call may have uncovered the full impact of stressful events which have built up past the point of personal control. The distress feels like a powerful reaction to just one call, but in reality, it may be a reaction to a long history of events. The focus of discussions, defusings, or debriefings is on relieving the pressure of both the recent and the old events.

When a person asks "Why am I reacting in this way to this call?" they are usually getting the first hint that the incident is stirring up memories or emotions. They may have been on hundreds of calls and suddenly one call overwhelms them. It is certainly something that makes a person wonder "Why?" "Why me?" "Why now?"

There is a considerable feeling of relief when a person is able to let go and get a traumatic event "off his chest." This relief will be apparent whether an event stands on its own or is just the last incident in a long history of distressing events. Talking things out initiates the recovery process. The latest research favors the concept that early support from a strong network of coworkers and friends is one of the most helpful things that can happen to a distressed person or a group of emergency workers.

Coworkers and other emergency personnel involved in the same call usually form a natural group that manifests trust, comfort, empathy, and concern for one another. That atmosphere allows for open expression of painful emotions and thoughts about a critical incident. Each member of the group, by talking about the incident, can encourage every other member to talk about their own experiences in the incident. Once the critical incident is talked out, the recovery process has been given a boost.

Some self-disclosure is essential for rapid emotional recovery. However, a word of caution is in order here. After a critical incident is discussed within the group of emergency workers, some personnel get the false impression that everyone, including their family members and friends outside emergency work, will want to listen to them with the same attention to detail and the same level of concern. This is not usually possible because those outside emergency work cannot have the same full understanding as those who are in it. Without that understanding they cannot react to the emergency worker with the same empathy and support that fellow emergency workers would provide. Even family members will listen carefully to the story of the critical incident, but they will be unable to have an exact understanding of the incident and all that happened at the scene. Their inability to comprehend the details of the event does not mean that they do not wish to be helpful or supportive or that they do not care. It simply means that without special training or personal experience they cannot fully appreciate the incident and its power to inflict distress on someone they love.

Most people who are not associated with emergency work will become uncomfortable if they hear in excessive detail about a painful critical incident. When emergency personnel try to relate to outsiders in the same manner that they would to each other in a defusing or debriefing session, they may end up feeling rejected. It is therefore important that they engage in self-disclosure selectively. Disclosure to fellow workers and loved ones is appropriate and generally helpful. But self-disclosure to others should be given only when it is in the best interests of the emergency person and the people who will hear it.[25]

PROFESSIONAL HELP

At times every effort we make to try to cope with and recover from stress ends in apparent failure. We begin to feel lost and out of control. Life becomes progressively more painful. Our health, job performance, happiness, and self-esteem all become jeopardized.

Those feelings may be signaling a need for outside assistance to help our own failing resources. It may be time to find a mental health professional. *It is advisable that the emergency person not wait until he or she is in a state of crisis before seeking outside support.* Recovery during a state of crisis is much more difficult to achieve because people do not think as clearly when in a crisis. Also, waiting too long may lengthen the time it takes for psychological support to work effectively. In other words, if the situation were such that one would normally respond to psychological support in about twelve sessions, excessive delay before going to seek help may extend the time required for effective psychological support to as many as 40 or 50 sessions.

Emergency personnel are notorious for delaying visits to medical doctors when they develop physical problems. They are far worse when it comes to their emotional needs. They continue to deny that they need help and assume that they are perfectly capable of dealing with the situation no matter how bad it is because they have always managed in the past. Chronic denial leads to a solidification of their problems. If they carry denial to an extreme, it may be impossible to reverse a bad situation. The ultimate cost is loss of career, family, friends, and happiness.

A person who is in a considerable amount of emotional pain may be unsure of the criteria on which they should judge their need for professional assistance. The most common criteria for deciding if a person needs professional assistance are as follows:

- Chronic sleep disturbance
- Chronic feelings of depression (sadness)
- Feeling generally unhappy
- Seriously declining job performance
- Troubled relationship with family
- Significant loss of interest in usual pursuits
- Withdrawal from contact with others
- Frequent loss of emotional control
- Frequent crying spells
- Frequent deep sighs
- Chronic anger/rage feelings
- Feeling lost/insecure/anxious/fearful
- Feeling paranoid

- Inability to stop thinking about painful issues
- Suicidal or homicidal thinking

Any person who is experiencing suicidal or homicidal thinking is in need of immediate intervention. He or she should be seen by a mental health professional as soon as possible. No one should take suicidal or homicidal thinking lightly. A life may be on the line and immediate action is necessary.[26]

A distressed person in need of professional support does not need all of the criteria cited above to seek out assistance; a few will do. If a person has four of these symptoms, they would probably benefit from some help. If they have eight or more, they certainly need help and should find a mental health professional as soon as possible.

A chronic problem that lasts from three months to a year or which repeats itself again and again over the course of a year or more is not going to go away by itself. Repetitive or chronic problems typically need professional intervention before they get resolved.

Choosing a Professional

There are many ways to find a professional to assist a person who feels the need for psychological support. The phone book is about the *worst* method to utilize to choose a mental health professional. Only by chance would a good one be picked. Considerably more caution should be exercised in choosing a professional to help you through a difficult problem. *Remember, the wrong kind of mental health support by the wrong mental health professional may be more damaging than no help at all.*

There are many differences in the training and experiences of mental health professionals. Specialties vary from person to person. Some do marriage and family counseling; some work with the seriously disturbed; others specialize in industrial psychology, children, forensic psychology, experimental psychology, the needs of women, and individual counseling.

It may be helpful to have some general information about what various mental health professionals do and the amount and type of training they have. Psychiatrists are medical doctors with special training in the workings of the human mind and the various abnormalities of the mind. They usually deal with the most seriously disturbed people. Some, however, prefer to work with marriages, families, and individuals in need of counseling. Psychiatrists may prescribe medications and perform other medical tasks to assist people with their problems.

Psychologists are not medical doctors. They cannot prescribe medications, nor can they perform other types of medical procedures. They receive master's degrees or Ph.D.'s. Many psychologists are skilled in administering and interpreting special diagnostic tests called psychological test batteries. In counseling they use techniques similar to those used by psychiatrists. They usually have specialties such as neuropsychology, industrial or medical psychology, family counseling, pediatrics, and individual counseling.

Social workers generally hold a master's degree. They tend to have special training in group and family work, although many have a preference for doing individual counseling. Social workers usually do not have training in administering and interpreting psychological tests. Social workers frequently work in hospitals, mental health centers, and clinics, although some work in private practices.

Psychiatric nurses also hold a master's degree and usually work within a hospital setting. Many tend to work on the psychiatric floor dealing with seriously disturbed people. However, there are some psychiatric nurses who prefer the private-practice office. They do not have the training, in most cases, to perform psychological tests. They cannot administer medication. Any medical procedures they might perform are limited to those which are allowed within their state and within the medical facilities in which they work.

Emergency personnel are not usually seriously mentally disturbed. They generally do not require the services of a psychiatrist. If they came to the office of another type of mental health professional, such as a psychologist, social worker, or psychiatric nurse, and were found to be seriously disturbed or if they needed specific type of assistance, they would be referred to a psychiatrist. Generally speaking, most emergency personnel obtain their assistance from psychologists or social workers.

Picking the right support person is not impossible; it just takes a little care to sort through the options. First, it is important to have a general definition of the problem (family, marriage, job, stress, grief, etc.) before seeking help. Then the task is to attempt to find a professional who has expertise in the area of the general problem. Several may need to be called and talked to briefly by phone before a choice is made. Sometimes it takes an office visit or two before a person feels confident in their choice. The last step is going for help and realizing that help depends on the ability of the emergency person to be open and honest in discussions with the professional and to be willing to stick to counseling long enough to give it a chance to work.

Guidelines for Choosing
a Mental Health Professional

Here are some additional guidelines that may be of use to emergency personnel seeking the assistance of a mental health professional:[27]

1. Do not approach professional help as if you were mentally deranged or "crazy." The vast majority of emergency personnel are not seriously disturbed and only need a little boost to get them over a difficult time. Normal people, like emergency personnel who seek out help when their own coping mechanisms are no longer working well, are showing wisdom and courage, not weakness and abnormalcy.

2. Ask a trusted friend if he or she knows of a good mental health professional. The best reference is usually from someone who may have used the services of a mental health professional.

3. If a friend does not know of a good mental health professional, the next best source for referral is a medical professional. They frequently have referred people in the past and have a pretty good idea who does what kind of work and how well they do it.

4. Hospital-based social workers are a very good source of referrals. Their job usually requires them to make a considerable number of referrals to other professionals. They know who handles which kinds of problems best.

5. College-based counseling services, community mental health centers, and employee assistance programs may also be able to provide names of a few people who do good counseling. They may be able to provide two or three names of mental health professionals in your area. That gives you a choice.

6. Check out the counselor, to make reasonably sure that you feel confident about him or her. A lack of confidence almost assures a failure of the counseling process. Ask questions! You are buying a professional service and you want to make sure that you are getting the best for you. Ask professionals what type and source of their training. What specialty areas do they claim? Do not be afraid to ask if they have had experience with your type of problem. Well-meaning but inexperienced mental health professionals are not in your best interests.

7. Work out all the administrative details in advance. Know about the costs and payment procedures, what is to be done in an emergency, and the usual meeting times. If the sessions are being covered by insurance, those details must be worked out in advance.

8. The helping process is a two-way street. It is not going to work if the counselor is expected to do all the work. The counselor should be looked upon as a coach. Much of the work is up to the person seeking help. The majority of people in counseling experience considerable relief after just a few sessions.

The real benefits of psychological support usually begin to show up by about the third month (twelve sessions). It will usually take longer than that to solidify the gains, so emergency workers are discouraged from leaving therapy too early. If positive changes do not show up in about twelve sessions, the counselor should be told and time should be allowed for changes to take place. If it is still not working, change therapists.

9. The therapist may be well trained, but he or she is not a mind reader. If a person does not open up and talk about the problem, there is no way for the therapist to know what is going on and what needs to be done to help.

10. No professional will attempt to engage a client in sexual activity. If it appears that the counselor is moving in that direction, it means that the counselor is not a true professional. Change therapists immediately and find one who lives up to the ethics and standards of the profession.

BEWARE OF FALSE CURES

The majority of this chapter has focused on the methods to help emergency personnel avoid acute, delayed, and especially cumulative stress. There are many techniques that people utilize which are counterproductive. The use of the techniques discussed below may turn a bad stress problem into a really serious one. They are false cures that usually do much more harm than good. Emergency personnel are urged to stay clear of these and choose more effective stress management techniques instead.

The most commonly utilized "false cure" among emergency people is alcohol. *Alcohol* directly enhances the stress response in the body, as described earlier. *People who have to use alcohol to cope better with their jobs have much more serious problems than the jobs themselves.*

The same comments can be applied equally well to other forms of *substance abuse.* Drugs of abuse always compound a stress condition. To cope effectively with stress, an emergency person needs a clear head. With drugs on board they are more likely to make errors in their attempts to cope. Their *resistance to stress is compromised.*

Freeze reactions, in which people become so fearful of becoming emotionally hurt that they will no longer take the risk of being close to others, have the danger of cutting off important sources of support from people in need of all the support they can get.

Avoidance techniques are also disruptive to emergency personnel. People cannot just go off somewhere and hide for the remainder of their lives. They must continue to live in a real world with real feelings and real threats. Getting help and getting back into life is a much healthier method of stress control.

Mind games, such as telling others that you are okay when you are not is another dangerous false cure. Honesty is certainly a more productive stress control method.

There are other false cures, but this list will get the main ideas across.

SUMMARY

In this chapter we emphasized the need for each person to accept his or her own responsibility for stress management. It was pointed out that organizations, although they have a vested interest in assisting their personnel to cope effectively with stress, could not be expected to actually perform all stress management tasks for their personnel. That responsibility is passed to individuals.

Emergency personnel were urged to adopt healthier life-styles. Better foods and better-balanced meals were suggested, and practical suggestions were made to reduce the intake of stress-producing foods. Personnel were also urged to increase their physical activity and to exercise more regularly to promote more-stress-reduced life-styles.

Other personal stress reduction items that were suggested included stopping smoking. Nicotine was described as a chemical that could directly enhance the stress reaction in a person. Emergency personnel were urged to engage in relaxation exercises, deep breathing, progressive muscle relaxation, and visual imagery.

The chapter concluded with useful information on spirituality, limited self-disclosure, and choosing a mental health professional when one's own resources become overwhelmed. Emergency personnel were encouraged to seek out help before their problems reached crisis proportions.

In the following two chapters we explore the types of support services that can be provided by well-trained Critical Incident Stress Debriefing teams. Such teams, which are being developed nationwide, have already been of great assistance in supporting emergency personnel before, during, and after they have been exposed to distressing situations.

REFERENCES

1. Girdano, D. A., and Everly, G. S. (1986). *Controlling Stress and Tension: A Holistic Approach* (2nd Ed.). Englewood Cliffs, NJ: Prentice-Hall.
2. Matteson, M. T., and Ivancevich, J. (1982). *Managing Job Stress and Health.* New York: Free Press.

3. Everly, G. S., and Rosenfeld, R. (1981). *The Nature and Treatment of the Stress Response: A Practical Guide for Clinicians*. New York: Plenum.

4. Gherman, E. M. (1981). *Stress and the Bottom Line: A Guide to Personal Well-Being and Corporate Health*. New York: AMACOM.

5. Hafen, B. Q. (1981). *How to Live Longer: Practical Ways You Can Beat Stress, Heart Disease, Cancer, Infection, and Chronic Illness*. Englewood Cliffs, NJ: Prentice-Hall.

6. Cox, T. (1978). *Stress*. Baltimore, MD: University Park Press.

7. Appelbaum, S. H. (1981). *Stress Management for Health Care Professionals*. Rockville, MD: Aspen Systems Corporation.

8. Smith, S. (1988). Food for fast times. *American West Airlines Magazine, 2*(12): 79–82.

9. Flynn, P. A. R. (1980). *Holistic Health: The Art and Science of Care*. Bowie, MD: R. J. Brady Co.

10. Brallier, L. (1982). *Successfully Managing Stress*. Los Altos, CA: National Nursing Review.

11. Eckholm, E., and Record, F. (1980). The affluent diet: A worldwide health hazard. In J. D. Adams (Ed.), *Understanding and Managing Stress: A Book of Readings*. La Jolla, CA: University Associates.

12. Everly, G. S., and Girdano, D. A. (1980). *The Stress Mess Solution*. Bowie, MD: R. J. Brady Co.

13. Monat, A., and Lazarus, R. S. (Eds.). (1985). *Stress and Coping: An Anthology* (2nd Ed.). New York: Columbia University Press.

14. Cooper, C. (1981). *The Stress Check*. Englewood Cliffs, NJ: Spectrum Books.

15. Everly, G. (1989). *A Clinical Guide to the Treatment of Human Stress*. New York: Plenum.

16. Solomon, R. (1987). Coping with vulnerability. Paper presented at the Third International Conference, "Stress, Helping the Helper," University of Maryland, Baltimore County.

17. Brown, W. D. (1983). *Welcome Stress! It Can Help You Be Your Best*. Minneapolis, MN: CompCare Publications.

18. Benson, H. (1975). *The Relaxation Response*. New York: Morrow.

19. Coutela, J. R., and Groden, J. (1978). *Relaxation*. Champaign, IL: Research Press.

20. Benson, H., Beary, J., and Carol, M. (1974). The "relaxation response." *Psychiatry, 37,* 37–46.

21. Jacobson, E. (1978). *You Must Relax*. New York: McGraw-Hill.

22. Gathel, R., and Price, K. (Eds.). (1979). *Clinical Applications of Biofeedback*. Oxford: Pergamon Press.

23. Basmajian, J., (Ed.). (1979). *Biofeedback: Principles and Practices for Clinicians*. Baltimore: Williams & Wilkins.

24. Sheehan, P. (1972). *The Function and Nature of Imagery.* New York: Academic Press.

25. Snyder, C. R., and Ford, C. E. (Eds.). (1987). *Coping with Negative Life Events: Clinical and Social Psychological Perspectives.* New York: Plenum.

26. Mitchell, J. T. (1986). By their own hand: suicide among emergency workers. *Chief Fire Executive, 2*(1): 48–52; 65; 72.

27. Mitchell, J. T. (1986). Where do I turn? Getting professional help. *Emergency Medical Services, The Journal of Emergency Care and Transportation, 15*(5): 57–58.

7

CRITICAL INCIDENT STRESS DEBRIEFING TEAM

In previous chapters we have pointed out that people who serve in the emergency services have unique jobs and are exposed to unique problems and stressors. They experience subtle, but often devastating effects from the services they provide to sick, injured, needy, distressed, threatened, or overwhelmed people. They do not avoid personal threats to themselves. Instead, they utilize their unique personalities to overcome incredible challenges. Their training, skills, experiences, and personalities combine to make them effective and efficient in accomplishing their individual or team missions. They are an uncommon breed compared to those who would not dare to have their jobs. Yet they remain ordinary people who are vulnerable to extraordinary stress in their work. Their personal, career, and physical lives may be "on the line."[1]

Efforts by people unfamiliar with the special personalities, operational procedures, stressors, and needs of emergency personnel to provide psychological support services will usually end in frustration and failure. Both the well-meaning but untrained support services provider and the emergency personnel who were the intended targets of the support will suffer from the failure to provide the right type of support at the right time by the right people.[2,3]

To assure emergency services organizations that the very best type of support services for emergency personnel is available in their localities, special psychological support teams are being developed nationwide and in some other countries as well. These teams, called Critical Incident Stress Debriefing teams, have been designed specifically to address the special personalities, job- and family-related stressors, and the support needs of emergency services personnel.[4] In this chapter we describe in considerable detail the major features and operations of a Critical Incident Stress Debriefing (CISD) team.

CISD TEAM OVERVIEW

The Critical Incident Stress Debriefing team is made up of a *partnership of mental health professionals* (master's degree or more in mental health) *and peer support personnel* who are drawn from the police, fire, emergency medical, nursing, dispatch, disaster management, and other emergency-oriented organizations. In addition, most CISD teams also invite selected members of the clergy to participate on the teams. The average CISD team has between twenty and forty members. About one-third of the membership are mental health professionals and the remainder are emergency personnel. From this pool of members a response team of four personnel are drawn to provide an actual debriefing. At least one of the CISD team members chosen to provide debriefing services must be a mental health professional, who serves as the team leader. The major purposes of CISD teams are to:

1. Prepare emergency personnel to manage their job-related stress
2. Assist emergency personnel who are experiencing the negative effects of stress after exposure to an unusually stressful event

The CISD team also serves in a number of different roles besides its *stress mitigation role* and its *critical incident stress recovery and assistance role*. The CISD team is active in *stress eduation and prevention programs* before a stressful event ever occurs. The CISD team serves as a *resource and referral network* for emergency personnel who need more support than can be provided by a debriefing. *Family education and support programs* are also an integral part of the team effort, as is the incorporation of CISD teams into the *disaster response* system.[4,5]

MULTIAGENCY, MULTIJURISDICTIONAL

The great majority of CISD teams serve in a voluntary (unpaid) multiagency and multijurisdictional approach. Generally, they provide services to police, firefighters, emergency medical personnel, nurses in emergency departments and critical care medicine, disaster response personnel, dispatchers, and others in emergency work. Since mental health professional resources are limited, it is best to have a *unified CISD* team which serves all of the emergency agencies in several jurisdictions. In addition, *except for the educational components of the program, it is dangerous for CISD team members to provide direct debriefing services to people who they know well and work with regularly. The emotional dangers of serving one's own people are considerable for both the helper and the person being helped. The practice of debriefing or providing defusing to one's own people should generally be avoided.* Finally, regional-based teams are more likely to be utilized more appropriately. They will avoid having members who are either under- or overused. Too little use on a CISD team leads to frustration and anger on the part of the members. The same reactions occur with excessive use of the team's resources.[6]

LEAD AGENCY

Every team needs a "lead agency," such as a fire department, police department, emergency medical services agency, or hospital to provide the resources necessary to assure a successful team. The lead agency provides a number of important services to the team. Those services include but are not limited to:[7]

- Funding for team development
- Coordinating team development
- Providing a team selection committee
- Providing the team coordinator
- Assisting in training the team
- Providing office space for team activities
- Providing administrative support services
- Assuring quality
- Providing training facilities
- Coordinating continuing education for the CISD team

It is important that agencies and individuals see the development of a CISD team as *only one step toward assisting emergency personnel.* The CISD team should transcend all political, jurisdictional, management versus line staff conflicts, union versus management issues, and other negative relationships between governmental and provider groups. *The CISD team must be as apolitical as possible to perform effectively its mission of helping emergency personnel.*[4]

Organizations and jurisdictions should not be engaged in conflict over which agency is going to run the CISD team. Instead, they should be promoting interagency and interjurisdictional cooperation and support for the team to assure the team's greatest success and a permanent existence. It sometimes takes a great deal for some agencies and jurisdictions to put aside their pride and go for the greater good. In the case of the CISD team, that is essential.

ASSURING CISD SUCCESS

A CISD team is generally created in an environment in which no or very few such services had previously been provided. Many of the emergency services people are unfamiliar with the concept of a CISD team and may resist its efforts out of ignorance of the process. Experience has demonstrated that three elements are essential if a team is to survive among the people it has been designed to serve.[4-7]

1. A successful CISD team must always provide training to all the emergency personnel in the jurisdiction. This training should address the basic elements of stress reduction and control before emergencies strike. Recruit classes and in-service programs need to be designed to provide stress management education to the providers. In addition, it is necessary to teach emergency people how to call upon and utilize the services of the CISD team before a crisis develops.

2. A successful CISD team depends heavily on team member cross training. Cross training means that mental health professionals ride along on fire, police, and emergency medical units or spend time in emergency rooms and dispatch centers before they begin to work with emergency services personnel. Emergency providers receive special training in crisis intervention skills, rapid assessment of stress reactions, human communication skills, and the procedures for making a referral for additional psychological services.

3. Meeting on a regular basis helps to assure the success of a CISD team. At the meetings, the members review the debriefings that have been provided. Quality issues are addressed. Also, team members receive additional training to ensure even better services for people in future debriefings. Mistakes are corrected, suggestions are presented, and personnel are given feedback on their debriefing activities. CISD meetings serve to air ideas about improving services and education for emergency personnel. They also provide a good chance for members to support one another in their own reactions to the privilege and pain of doing debriefings. Finally, CISD meetings may serve a social function for the members, who do such important and demanding work.

To be successful, a CISD team should also keep in mind the following important guidelines. These guidelines were developed to enhance a team's ability to do its job while avoiding significant problems from legal and operational points of view.[8]

- *Teams should not charge* individuals who attend debriefings fees for services. Most teams provide free services for defusings and debriefings. This guideline helps to keep the situation clear of the fears and anxieties associated with money issues and psychological services. Those who provided the services through which they were stressed are often working voluntarily. They resent the concept that they would be charged as individuals to recover from situations they were traumatized by when they freely offered their services to their communities.
- Individuals who attend a debriefing must always be granted the *right to refuse to talk* about the critical incident if they choose.
- Individuals and groups must always be guaranteed that their right to *strict confidentiality* will be maintained.
- *The Critical Incident Stress Debriefing process should be adhered to* during a debriefing. Variations from the model may disrupt the flow of the process and have a greater chance of producing errors.
- *Advice from the CISD team members must always be well thought out,* appropriate, prudent, and as proven a stress reduction technique as possible.

TEAM MEMBERS

Clinical Director

The clinical director is the overall leader of a CISD team who has the responsibility for assuring quality services of the team. The clinical director is usually a high-ranking mental health professional who has a sincere interest in the debriefing team and its work. The clinical director provides the following:[7,8]

- General supervision of the CISD team's mental health professionals
- Assurance that quality continuing education programs are provided to team members
- Review and monitoring of debriefings
- Assistance in establishing cross training for team members
- Representation for the team before public, governmental, and other agencies
- Assistance in developing team-written operational protocols
- Assistance in choosing team members

- Assistance in referrals and follow-up services
- Clinical support and program guidance to the team coordinator and members

CISD Team Coordinator

The team coordinator position is among the most important on the team. It is certainly the busiest. The tasks of the team coordinator are so varied and plentiful that the position is often shared by two or even three CISD coordinators. The coordinator is responsible for the phone calls and other coordination efforts that are necessary to dispatch a CISD team for a debriefing. In addition, the coordinator is responsible for day-to-day operation of the team. The position is best filled by a peer support member of the team. The coordinator does the following:[7,8]

- Manages the CISD team
- Recruits new members
- Assists in team member selection
- Assists in the educational activities of the team
- Answers requests for CISD information
- Evaluates requests for debriefings
- Seeks guidance from the clinical director on unusual situations
- Dispatches the team
- Organizes team meetings
- Establishes committees
- Maintains team records
- Maintains the referral list
- Teaches stress programs to emergency personnel
- Keeps up with current research, experiences, and theories related to emergency services stress, etc.
- Maintains an active stance in the international CISD network
- Performs other duties as necessary on behalf of the team

Team Liaison

The primary responsibility of the team liaison is to represent the interests of the team before the lead agency. Team liaison officers make sure that the CISD team obtains from the lead agency whatever support it needs to perform its work. This might include such items as telephone services, file cabinets, office supplies, and postage. The team liaison person should be of sufficient rank within the lead agency to assure that the legitimate requests of the team are not ignored or unnecessarily delayed.[7,8]

Mental Health Professionals

The mental health professionals (often called professional support personnel) on the team work as the team leaders or co-leaders during an actual debriefing. They also assist in training and supervision of peer support team members. Mental health professionals help team members by providing psychological support for other team members when a debriefing has dealt with material so intense that the debriefers may need to talk about their own reactions to the debriefing. Many make themselves available for individual referrals if they happen to be in private practice or in an agency that is able to provide clinical services. Of course, once individual referrals are made to a mental health professional, the usual fees and other requirements may be applicable since the services at that point are beyond the debriefing process. Professional support members of a CISD team also perform many of the following duties:[9]

- Assist with the team's educational activities
- Assist in the development of referral sources
- Provide the minimal necessary paperwork to the team coordinator
- Assist the coordinator in determining the appropriateness of a debriefing request
- Facilitate the debriefing process
- Provide follow-up contacts to individuals and groups after the debriefing
- Etc.

Peer Support Personnel

Peer support personnel are chosen from the emergency services. They are police officers, firefighters, emergency medical technicians, paramedics, nurses, dispatchers, disaster response personnel, and other emergency workers. They are chosen because they have the respect of a large majority of their peers, are mature, care about the well-being of their fellow emergency workers, understand how destructive uncontrolled stress might be, and want to help people deal with and conquer stress. Peer support personnel also perform the following:[7,9]

- Initiate the first contacts with those who have responded to the scene of a critical incident
- Assess the need for defusings or debriefings
- Contact the CISD coordinator to begin the process of setting up a debriefing
- Perform defusings under the supervision of the mental health professionals on the team

- Provide on-scene support services (psychological first aid) as necessary
- Call for mental health support when their training and resources are exceeded
- Assist in CISD team educational activities
- Etc.

CRITICAL INCIDENTS

Critical incidents are any events that have sufficient emotional power to overcome the usual coping abilities of emergency personnel who are exposed to them. Some of them were mentioned in Chapter 2, but a brief review of some of the more common critical incidents will be helpful. The typical critical incidents capable of causing distress for emergency personnel are:[5,10]

- Line-of-duty death
- Serious injury to emergency personnel
- Serious multiple-casualty incident
- Suicide of an emergency person
- Traumatic deaths of children
- Serious injuries to children
- Events with excessive media interest
- Victims known to the emergency person
- An event that has an unusually powerful impact on the personnel

Defusings and debriefings can be powerful processes that have great potential to prevent serious stress reactions from becoming extremely damaging to emergency personnel. They have frequently accelerated the recovery process. However, if they are overused, that is, if they are utilized for routine events, defusings and debriefings can be diluted and their power sustantially reduced. *It is very important that defusings and debriefings not be overused. They should be reserved for events that have extraordinary power to negatively affect emergency personnel.*

ON-SCENE SUPPORT SERVICES

Peer support personnel play a key role in providing on-scene support services to distressed emergency responders. They usually arrive at the scene with the primary goal of performing their usual emergency job. However, when they notice an obviously distressed coworker, they may temporarily turn their attention toward that person and render assistance until the distress lessens. Their actions on behalf of their coworkers must be approved by command staff so that operations in the field are not disrupted. Generally, the assistance rendered to coworkers is limited and brief. For example, a distressed responder may be moved fifty feet from the extrication zone to reduce the auditory and visual stimuli that are causing the distress. As soon as possible, peer support personnel are expected to conclude their assistance and return to their usual duties. There are generally three things that peer support personnel may handle at the scene:

1. Brief assistance to *obviously distressed* coworkers, as described above.
2. *Advice to the command* staff as the situation warrants.
3. Brief assistance to victims and their family members to reduce interference with operations. Once other appropriate victim-oriented agencies arrive, the care of distressed victims is turned over to the qualified agencies.

To provide the right kind of support services in the field, peers need additional training from mental health professionals on an ongoing basis. Regular attendance at CISD team meetings assures that peers are given opportunities to improve their skills.[11]

DEMOBILIZATION SERVICES

This intervention is reserved for a large-scale event. A large-scale event usually has about 50 percent or more of the forces from a particular sector involved in emergency operations for a considerable period of time. Most large-scale events last longer than eight hours. Demobilizations take place at a demobilization center away from the scene. Personnel are ordered to the center when their work at the scene is completed. The entire process lasts a total of 30 minutes. Ten minutes are used in giving stress information; 20 minutes are allocated to feeding and resting the crews. The demobilization center allows several important things to happen.[7,8]

• Personnel are given information about stress and the typical signs and symptoms that people experience. They are also advised about the best methods to deal with stress reactions should they occur. Personnel are told that some people have little or no reaction to a significantly stressful event, whereas others have considerable reactions. Stress-related handout sheets are distributed at the end of the session.

- The demobilization center provides a place where emergency workers can rest, eat, and get fluids into their system in a comfortable environment before they return to their quarters, go back in service, or are released to their homes.

- The demobilization center also provides a good place for command staff to make announcements and to thank personnel for their work. Frequently updates on the condition of injured personnel are given.

- Many demobilization centers allow an initial ventilation of feelings on an individual or group basis, but only if the personnel wish to open up about the situation and their reactions. Otherwise, their right to silence is respected.

- Some personnel may be found to have special needs. These should be addressed by the professional support staff with the approval of the commanders of the organization.

DEFUSINGS

Defusings are a much shorter, less formal, and less structured version of Critical Incident Stress Debriefing. They are given within a few hours of the event. Usually, anywhere from one to four hours after an event is ideal. If they are not given within twelve hours, the window of opportunity is lost and they are not given at all. In that case a formal debriefing may be necessary. The key to successful reduction of emergency services stress is rapid intervention.

Defusings last about 30 to 45 minutes. They are typically managed by peer support personnel but may be led by a mental health person if the peer decides that that is necessary. The main purpose is to stabilize the working crew so that they can be returned to normal service or allowed to go home without unusual stress if they are at the end of their shift. In some cases, personnel may not be able to finish a shift because of intense stress. Alternatives to continued work may need to be found. Command staff must approve of any unusual decisions that would affect staffing of the unit. The defusing is a small-group process and the personnel of a particular unit at the scene are brought together. Unlike the formal debriefing, which includes all personnel involved in the incident, defusing concentrates on the most seriously affected workers—usually a police officer and partner, an engine or truck company, or an ambulance crew.

Defusing allows for a little initial ventilation of the reactions to the event. It also provides stress-related information to the addressed crew. Handouts may be used if they have been developed and stocked in advance. Usually, defusing will accomplish one or two major goals in reference to the formal debriefing process. *A well-run defusing will either eliminate the need to provide a formal debriefing, or it will enhance the formal debriefing.*[7,8]

CRITICAL INCIDENT STRESS DEBRIEFINGS

Critical Incident Stress Debriefings are structured group meetings that emphasize ventilation of emotions and other reactions to a critical event. In addition, they emphasize educational and informational elements which are of great assistance for emergency personnel in understanding and dealing with the stress generated by the event. Critical Incident Stress Debriefings are essentially discussions of the critical incident in confidential meetings. They are not considered psychotherapy, nor are they psychological treatment. Instead, debriefings are discussions designed to put a bad situation into perspective. The two major goals of debriefings are to reduce the impact of a critical event and to accelerate the normal recovery of normal people who are suffering through normal but painful reactions to abnormal events.[4-6]

CISDs have many benefits. They provide a chance to ventilate pent-up feelings. They also provide opportunities for stress reduction education, emotional reassurance, and forewarning personnel what signs and symptoms of distress might materialize later. Debriefings usually reduce the fallacy of uniqueness and abnormality. CISDs are a positive interaction with mental health professionals. They enhance group cohesiveness, interagency cooperation, and serve as an opportunity for screening and referral. Debriefings are considered a good stress prevention method.[12]

Deciding to Provide a Debriefing

There are a number of criteria on which peer support personnel and command staff might decide to provide a CISD to personnel after a critical incident.[13]

- Many individuals within a group appear to be distressed after a call.
- The signals of distress appear to be quite severe.
- Personnel demonstrate numerous behavioral changes.
- Personnel make significant errors on calls occurring after the critical incident.
- Personnel request help.
- The event is extraordinary.

- Various agencies are showing the same reactions.
- Signals of distress continue beyond three weeks.

Important CISD Considerations

The formal CISD process achieves its best effects when it is offered after 24 hours and before 72 hours following a critical incident. The CISD is led by a mental health professional and several peer support personnel. The typical debriefing usually lasts three hours. It is held in a room which has movable furniture so that the seats can be arranged in a circle. Note taking, recorders, and media personnel are forbidden. Personnel must be relieved of response duties for new calls. Radios should be off.

Pre-debriefing Activities

Prior to a CISD, all the coordination elements must be in place. The debriefing must be announced to those involved. The room must be selected; the time is set; refreshments are arranged for the end of the debriefing; the command staff makes arrangements to have the unit's calls managed by other departments or by personnel not involved in the incident.

The four-member CISD team (its usual size) will generally arrive about 45 minutes early. The team members have three important tasks to accomplish in the time before the debriefing. First, they will review the photographs, newspaper articles, videotapes, and incident report. Next they will want to meet casually some of the personnel who are gathering at the debriefing center. Finally, CISD team members will want to have a brief strategy meeting before beginning the debriefing.

CISD Process

Introduction

The introduction phase of a debriefing is the time in which the team leader gradually introduces the process, encourages participation by the group, and sets the ground rules by which the debriefing will work. There are many things that need to be said to the group before it begins the CISD. The participants are told:[10-14]

1. That the entire process is confidential and that every one is urged to maintain a pact of confidentiality with one another regarding whatever is said during the session.
2. That they do not have to speak if they choose not to but, they are encouraged to discuss the event.

3. That no breaks are taken but that personnel may leave to attend to their personal needs and then return to the room. They are told that leaving before the end of the session might endanger their recovery because many things will be unresolved.

4. That every person is asked to speak only for himself or herself and for no one else.

5. That they do not need to get into detail which could jeopardize an investigation or cause any person in the debriefing difficulties on the job.

6. That pagers are to be turned off.

7. That all personnel are equal during the debriefing. No one has rank during the debriefing.

8. That the CISD is not part of an investigation nor is it a critique of the incident but that it is a group discussion to assure that the personnel are going to make as quick a recovery as possible.

9. That the CISD team member will be available after the debriefing if someone wants to talk individually. People are encouraged to ask questions of the team during the debriefing.

10. That with some exceptions that arise on a case-by-case basis, people who were not involved in the incident are not allowed in the debriefing.

11. (Additional comments are added on a case-by-case basis depending on the needs of the group.)

The Fact Phase

During this phase, the group is asked to describe briefly their job during the incident and from their own perspective, some facts regarding what happened. This is a relatively easy phase for most people since the facts are almost always easier to discuss than a person's reactions to an event. The fact phase recreates the event for the CISD attendees.

It is understood that talking about the facts of an event may be uncomfortable. But the great benefit is that once something gets talked about openly, the participants feel a sense of power in eventually being able to overcome the situation and not be defeated by it. Keeping things inside oneself leads to the development of a number of painful emotions which are frequently unnecessary and destructive to the person. People who keep things inside themselves feel more unique and abnormal than do those who are willing to discuss the incident.

The Thought Phase

The CISD leader asks the members of the group to discuss their first thought during the stressful event. This helps the CISD process to tap into the more personal aspects of the situation. The personal thoughts often get hidden behind the facts and bringing them out into the open affirms that one's own thoughts are important and not to be forgotten and buried beneath the facts of the situation.

The Reaction Phase

The reaction phase is designed to move the group participants from the predominantly cognitive level of intellectual processing into the emotional level of processing. This does *not* mean that everyone is going to cry. It just means that in human beings experiences are processed on two levels—the cognitive and the emotional. The cognitive process is what we think and the emotional level is what we feel. Only a person out of touch with themselves would think that they have no feelings about their experiences. They may not talk about them all the time, but they do have them. Human beings who function on both the cognitive and the emotional levels are usually healthier and happier. Those who ignore the emotional level of function often end up with stress-related diseases. Since one of the objects of the CISD is to prevent the development of stress-related diseases, it goes into both the cognitive and emotional levels of processing experiences. The CISD, in essence, encourages people to be whole and not to review their experiences in a cognitive vacuum void of human emotions.

The typical question that moves people from the cognitive to the emotional level of processing is: "What was the worse thing about the event?" It is surprising what complex statements from the CISD group participants such a question can trigger. Most CISD groups come out of this portion of the debriefing believing that it is okay for them to have not only their thoughts about an experience but their feelings as well.

The Symptom Phase

The symptom phase begins the movement back from the predominantly emotional processing levels toward the cognitive processing levels. It serves as a transition phase much like the thought phase described earlier. In the symptom phase, the CISD participants are asked to describe their cognitive, physical, emotional, and behavioral signs and symptoms or signals of distress which appeared:

- At the scene or within a 24-hour period
- A few days after the event
- Are still being experienced at the time of the debriefing

The Teaching Phase

Once the signals of distress have been discussed, the CISD team members begin to relay information regarding stress reactions and what can be done to alleviate them. A good starting point is to tell the group that the signals of distress they have encountered are normal and that they will generally subside over time. Whenever possible, specific instructions for stress reduction are given. The group is also given other pertinent information regarding stress reactions and recovery from a stressful situation. Questions are invited from the group. The object of the teaching phase of the CISD is to provide the participants with as much information as they might need to overcome their stress. Sometimes, specific instructions are given for the care of their children. At other times it is necessary to give them information on the grief process, suicide, pediatrics, AIDS, the normal physiological responses to stress, or any other topic which would arm them with knowledge by which they can better control their stress.

The Reentry Phase

This is the wrap-up phase, in which any additional statements or questions can be presented by the group. Sometimes it is necessary for the CISD team to state things that people could not or would not say during the debriefing, such as feelings that were too difficult to verbalize. Anything that the participants have not said or any repetition of previously stated material is encouraged.

Sometimes the members of the group decide to formulate some sort of supportive contract with one another. At other times they decide to do something as a group to assist others. Occasionally, the group decides that it needs additional information and plans an information-gathering project or educational project. The idea is that doing something as a group gives people a sense of power and control.

There are times when no group activity or contract evolves out of a debriefing. It is not a necessary conclusion to a CISD. It is up to the group, not the CISD team.

During the latter stages of this segment, the CISD team members are required to make a summary statement to the group. No one else has to speak if they do not wish to do so. The invitation is made, but no one is forced to speak. Handouts with phone numbers of the CISD team members should be distributed at each debriefing. Writing phone numbers on a board is *not* a good idea. People are often too embarrassed to copy those down.

Figure 7–1 depicts the CISD process from the cognitive levels of processing through the emotional levels and back again to the cognitive levels.

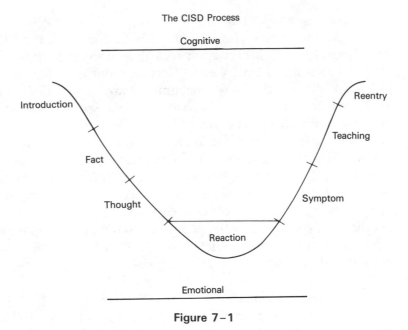

Figure 7-1

Post-debriefing Activities/Meeting

Immediately after the debriefing concludes, CISD team members will make themselves available to the group for individual contacts, additional questions, requests for referrals, personal reassurance, and so on. In addition, CISD team members seek out those who may be having the most difficulty and attempt to give them reassurance, instructions, advice, referrals, and so on. This activity has been known to go on for an hour or more after the session, but those who must leave can certainly do so.

The last step is for the debriefers to meet on the way home and discuss among themselves the debriefing that just ended. They decide what steps may be necessary for follow-up purposes. They critique their performance with the intention of correcting their mistakes and providing an improved debriefing process to the next group. They also give credit for alertness— for example, for catching what one person said and reacting to it. But more important than anything else is the fact that a debriefing is a powerful experience for the debriefing team as well. They need to talk about how the debriefing affected them. They need to get their emotions out in the open before they go home and feel depressed. Debriefers need support as well, and they get it from one another.[7,8]

Follow-Up Services

Follow-up services are extremely important. They usually begin within twenty-four hours of the debriefing. Telephone calls are made, requests for referrals are fulfilled, individuals or groups may be checked on, additional printed material is mailed, visits to the station may be arranged, and command officers are given *general* advice about how best to care for their distressed personnel. (Absolutely nothing is said to a command officer that would violate confidential material shared by the group during the debriefing.) In some instance a second debriefing may be necessary. Also, individuals or small groups might need additional support.[7,8,14]

Consideration should be made for anniversary dates, which are usually hard times, and for evaluations later in the year.

Individual Consultations

When only one, two, or three persons are affected by a critical incident and everyone else is just fine, group debriefings are not provided. Instead, the individuals are seen one at a time or in a very small group. Bringing an entire crew or squad together for a debriefing when only two or three of their members were affected by an incident will cause a great deal of anger and frustration in the emergency personnel.[5]

Specialty Debriefing

On occasion a nonemergency group with no other readily available resources, such as disaster victims, school students, or industrial groups, may request a debriefing from a CISD team. These requests are filled on a case-by-case basis. The criteria for doing a specialty debriefing should include some of the following:[4-6]

- The magnitude of the event is overwhelming.
- Other resources are not readily available.
- Emergency services personnel will not be without services because a debriefing is given to an outside group.
- Humanitarian reasons.

Significant Other Support

Some incidents are so disruptive that the loved ones of emergency personnel may need *separate* debriefings. A serious injury or line-of-duty death incident is a good example; without support the loved ones may suffer excessively.

SUMMARY

This chapter was devoted entirely to the activities of a Critical Incident Stress Debriefing team because it is such an important factor in assisting emergency personnel with their stress. CISD teams have direct benefits for the personnel who go through the education programs and the debriefings. They also have many hidden benefits, such as the positive influence they exert over the emergency services to provide stress reduction and control programs as part of the organizational strategy of maintaining healthy personnel.

It is believed that an effective CISD program may be one of the many steps necessary to assure that good emergency workers, who have seen a few too many painful scenes, are not unnecessarily lost from the systems that use their services. CISD programs go a long way to assure that the health, safety, and performance of emergency responders will remain at its peak.

REFERENCES

1. Graham, N. K. (1981). Done in, fed up, burned out: Too much attrition in EMS. *Journal of Emergency Medical Services, 6*(1): 24–29.
2. Graham, N. K. (1981). How to avoid a short career. *Journal of Emergency Medical Services 6*(2): 25–31.
3. Raphael, B. (1986). *When Disaster Strikes: How Individuals and Communities Cope with Catastrophe.* New York: Basic Books.
4. Mitchell, J. T. (1986). Teaming up against critical incident stress. *Chief Fire Executive, 1*(1): 24; 36; 84.
5. Mitchell, J. T. (1983). When disaster strikes; The critical incident stress debriefing process. *Journal of Emergency Medical Services, 8*(1): 36–39.
6. Mitchell, J. T. (1983). Guidelines for psychological debriefings. *Emergency Management Course Manual.* Emmitsburg, MD: Federal Emergency Management Agency, Emergency Management Institute.
7. Kennedy-Ewing, L. (1988). *Delaware County Critical Incident Stress Management Program.* Media, PA: Delaware County Department of Human Resources.
8. Tritt, P. (1984). *Mayflower (Denver) Critical Incident Stress Debriefing Team Protocols.* Denver, Colorado: Swedish Hospital System, Paramedic Training Program.

9. Mitchell, J. T. (1986). Critical incident stress management. *Response,* Sept./ Oct., 24–25.

10. Mitchell, J. T. (1984). Strategies for coping in a charged environment: High tension keeping stress under control. *Firehouse, 9*(9), 86–88, 90.

11. Mitchell, J. T. (1987). Effective stress control at major incident. *Maryland Fire and Rescue Bulletin, 15*(6): 3; 6.

12. Mitchell, J. T. (1985). Healing the helper. In B. Greene (Ed.) *Role Stressors and Supports for Emergency Workers.* Washington, DC: Center for Mental Health Studies of Emergencies, U.S. Department of Health and Human Services.

13. Mitchell, J. T. (1987). The impact of stress on emergency service personnel policy issues in emergency response. In L. K. Comfort (Ed.). *Managing Disaster.* Durham, NC: Duke University Press.

14. Hartsough, D. M., and Garaventa Myers, D. *Disaster Work and Mental Health: Prevention and Control of Stress among Workers.* Washington, DC: Center for Mental Health Studies of Emergencies, U.S. Department of Health and Human Services.

8

STRESS CONTROL MODEL
FOR EMERGENCY SERVICES

8

Stress has been identified in previous chapters as a major concern for those interested in maintaining the quality of service and quality of life for emergency responders. In this chapter we present a unified model that describes the most helpful steps for stress reduction interventions. The stress reduction model presented here defines a sequence of steps for stress intervention and then details the skills, knowledge, and attitudes that are essential to implement the model. The *reaper* model evolved out of emergency experience. It is a way of conceptualizing an effective strategy to reduce emergency services stress.

When an organization decides to address the issue of stress systematically, a decision model should be developed as part of standard operating policies and procedures. Establishing these policies removes the question of *whether* to have a response for stressful situations and replaces it with a guide for the type or level of intervention.

The Reaper model is composed of six levels of intervention. Each letter in the name "Reaper" stands for a significant term associated with a specific level of response to the stress problem in emergency services. The model looks like this:

R - Recognize
E - Educate
A - Accept
P - Permit
E - Explore
R - Refer

Any phase of the model can be developed separately, but it is most beneficial for emergency providers if the program is implemented from beginning to end. Implementation of the Reaper model for stress reduction demands an organizational commitment of time, effort, and resources. Without that organizational commitment and the dedication of the organization's leadership, efforts to reduce stress will meet with failure.[1]

RECOGNIZE
e
a
p
e
r

Stress is a reality and we must learn not only to cope with the pressure of emergency work but to use stress to help us achieve a higher quality of professional and personal life. A comprehensive stress awareness program requires that we not only identify and understand *distress* in our lives, but that we become more active and devote attention to the *eustress* or the positive, creative forms of stress (see Chapter 1). The physical, mental, and emotional changes associated with the stress response are all designed to help us in some way. It is only when we fail to recognize and utilize these changes in a positive way that we give in to the destructive components of stress.

When we understand the logical outcomes associated with the stress response, we can use stress to our advantage. We manipulate the outcome to best suit our purposes and in doing so, allow the stress response to complete a normal process for which it is designed—protecting the body and mind from destruction. The stress response did not evolve to kill us; rather, it acts to help us cope with a wide variety of situations that we perceive to be threatening, challenging, or involving significant change.[2-3]

Unfortunately, such comments as "Stress is just part of the job and if it bothers you, get out!" or "We never had programs like this in the past, so why do we have them now?" are still heard from people who do not regard stress as a major concern for emergency responders. If there is no awareness that a significant problem exists, there will be little or no planning to help those suffering from the destructive effects of emergency services stress. During the phase termed *recognize,* emphasis is placed on:[4]

1. The identification of stress as a normal process associated with emergency work

2. The development of intervention techniques to utilize the stress response in a beneficial way

3. Implementing techniques to inhibit the stress process when a destructive level of stress is encountered

4. Preventing as much distress as possible through proactive planning, wellness-oriented programs, and broad-based physical, mental, and social support systems.

It is important for those in command positions to recognize the signs and symptoms of stress in responders. The key to recognizing the changes that stress creates is to *know your personnel*. Anyone can memorize the lists of changes associated with stress, but these lists are of little value unless the command person knows the characteristic behaviors of each person in the unit. When stress-related changes occur, they are easier to recognize if the command staff members know their people and if they are sensitive to *significant behavior changes in their personnel*.

r
EDUCATE
a
p
e
r

Once stress is acknowledged by the emergency community, the organizations are ready for the next level of intervention education. The education component is broken down into five phases of training.

Phase 1

Phase 1 programs are for the front-line emergency responders. These programs provide six to eight hours of training on such topics as: orientation to stress; the impact of stress on mental, physical, and emotional function; emergency services stress; intervention techniques for individual response to stress; and networking to develop a personal support system. Phase 1 is therefore a general overview of stress and stress management techniques for emergency personnel.

Phase 2

Phase 2 programs are for emergency officers, supervisors, or administrators. As in phase 1, this phase includes a basic review of stress. This review provides consistency in terminology, concepts, and principles and is designed to facilitate the communications process at all levels of instruction and organizational intervention.

Phase 2 provides managers with an opportunity to develop skills and strategies for the stress-related problems presented to them by emergency responders. Topics reviewed in phase 2 include: recognition of stress signs and symptoms, effective human communications, conflict resolution, team building, effective leadership, making referrals, and an orientation to Critical Incident Stress Debriefing.

These topics do provide a general overview and working knowledge of many management principles, but they are not designed as a substitute for professional development in management theory, issues of command, incident command, or personnel administration. Phase 2 programs require six to eight hours for completion.

Phase 3

Phase 3 addresses the concerns of emergency workers and their families regarding the impact of emergency services stress on the family. Programs based on such topics as "Emergency Stress and the Family" are designed to help families understand their behavior as a response to stress brought about by emergency work. Topics covered in a phase 3 program include: an orientation to stress; the personality types of emergency personnel; the family as a system; human communications in the family system; problem solving; rebuilding relationships; and intimacy.

Families provide the major support system for emergency providers, and thus increased attention should be focused on family needs, roles, and values in both supporting and gaining support from emergency personnel. Phase 3 programs are three to four hours in length and are frequently presented in the evenings. Spouses and emergency providers are encouraged to attend together.[5]

Phase 4

Phase 4 programs are designed for emergency personnel who desire to become peer support personnel on a CISD team (see Chapter 7). Peer support is a vital component of the debriefing process. Their firsthand knowledge of emergency operations provides a credible link between the debriefing team and the responders during a debriefing. Because of the critical nature of their role, prospective peer support personnel should be screened before being accepted on a critical incident stress team. Peer support personnel are required to complete an application for the CISD team. They are asked to participate in a screening process which includes:

- A personal history or résumé
- Response to a number of questions that tap into one's personal goals and motivations
- A psychological screening profile
- Two letters of recommendation (one from a commander)
- A personal interview with a CISD team member screening committee

Phase 4 programs include: an orientation to stress, the recognition and impact of acute stress, group dynamics, the helping process, communication, the rationale and process for debriefing, defusing, and one-on-one emotional support.

Phase 4 programs require a minimum of sixteen hours of initial training and follow-up sessions with mental health professionals to enhance the basic skills learned during the orientation training session. Follow-up sessions may take place in the context of CISD team meetings which are held regularly (usually every four to six weeks) after the team is formed.[6]

Phase 5

Phase 5 is designed for mental health professionals who have expressed an interest in becoming debriefing team members. Participants are screened prior to placement on a team through individual interviews with the CISD team screening committee.

The program for mental health professionals is designed to orient them to the unique needs of emergency responders. Topics presented during phase 5 include an orientation to emergency services stress, an orientation to general stress, the personality characteristics of emergency personnel, the debriefing process, the roles of debriefing team members, and the function and value of mental health professionals as debriefing team members. These programs are six to sixteen hours in length. They are often given jointly with the peer support personnel so that they have an opportunity to meet each other. Subsequent training is provided by means of field experiences as observers on emergency units.

Both the *recognize* and *educate* aspects of the Reaper model are primarily preventive. Each is designed to prevent or minimize the occurrence of significant trauma following either a specific, intense event or the accumulation of destructive changes through exposure to chronically stressful situations. The next level of intervention, *accept*, is the first one in which direct interpersonal contact occurs as a result of stress.

r
e
ACCEPT
p
e
r

When the behaviors or symptoms associated with distress appear, they create personal concern, if we are the stressed person, or others who exhibit the symptoms. Emergency responders are helpful by nature, so there is an inherent desire to respond to the perceived needs of any person in distress, and this drive is enhanced if the person happens to be a member of the emergency services. Often the desire to help is blocked by a lack of information on how to help or a lack of skill and experience in the helping process. The *recognize* and *educate* aspects of the Reaper model provide the basic information needed to help. The *accept* aspect provides the mechanism and skill to apply the information.

The *accept* intervention process usually occurs one-on-one or in small-group interventions. This type of meeting frequently occurs immediately after a call that has been difficult or emotionally distressing. The meeting may be referred to as a "defusing" if it is for a small group or an "individual consultation" if it is for a person. Both defusings and individual consultations provide an excellent opportunity for command personnel or peer support personnel to assess the impact of the call on the responders. The assessment might indicate the need for further intervention, such as a debriefing to help the emergency personnel cope with the emotional trauma of the call. It may also clarify that no further assistance is necessary.[7]

The defusing or consultations also give responders an opportunity to assess how their fellow team members are handling their reactions to a difficult situation, as well as an opportunity to deal with their own feelings about the call. If the call was prolonged or exceptionally difficult, it might be helpful to request a mental health professional to help the peer support person with the defusing process, but in most cases an outside professional support person is not necessary. The defusing session gives an opportunity for those within a close knit team to help each other. The warmth, compassion, trust, and empathy expressed by team members for each other provides a nurturing environment that facilitates the emotional healing process.

There are various types of statements that can help other emergency personnel. A key element of the *accept* process is empathy. An expression of empathetic support, such as "I can understand the feelings you are expressing," focuses on the present, emotional healing, and personal power, whereas a sympathetic expression such as "I feel sorry for you," focuses on the past, loss, and helplessness. There are times when the expression of sympathy is correct and appropriate (an aid in the grieving and mourning process), but for the emotional support needed to adapt in a healthy way to the stresses of emergency services, empathy is more appropriate. Most peer support personnel need additional human communications skills training to function better in the task of providing emotional support to their peers during a period of intense stress.

There will be occasions when a call has been much broader in scope and had involved such powerful emotional trauma on the emergency services groups that a more intensive response is required. During the fourth level of the Reaper model, *permission,* special interventions are initiated that will address the group and individual needs evolving out of a powerful critical incident.

r
e
a
PERMISSION
e
r

Permission to deal openly with the feelings that follow a critical incident is given when an organization endorses any level of psychological support. It is not enough, though, to give consent for a formalized group response following an incident. The department, agency, or company needs to provide aggressive leadership in securing the appropriate levels of emotional support needed by emergency responders. Line personnel take their cues from their leaders. They quickly perceive half-hearted or insincere gesture which are produced for show and not for substance.[8]

Permission is an intervention that not only allows the expression of feelings about an event, but actually encourages the expression of those reactions. The substance of the permission level of intervention in the Reaper model is found in the educational and psychological support called the Critical Incident Stress Debriefing (see Chapter 7). It is usually scheduled 24 to 72 hours after the incident. The CISD is a meeting in which people are openly encouraged to discuss the experiences, feelings, reactions, and impact associated with a major incident.

A debriefing is not without psychological hazards. To ensure the safety of all participants, the debriefing team is composed of at least one mental health professional (who holds at least a master's degree) as well as specially trained peer support personnel. It is important not to confuse or mix the CISD together with the operations critique. The two are separate in goals, orientation, techniques, and outcomes. (See Chapter 7 for a detailed description of the defusing and debriefing processes.)

After the debriefing some responders may require further assistance to cope with a specific incident or the cumulative stressors of emergency service. The emergency organization needs to be responsive to these needs and develop structured interventions that help members cope with their stress. Organizational interventions are defined within the *explore* level (see also Chapter 5).

r
e
a
p
EXPLORE
r

As professionals, whether career or volunteer, we have always maintained that we take care of our own. In a very real sense, we are like a family. When it is recognized that a person is in trouble, we call on all our resources to help that person.

The *explore* intervention is one where we help a person clearly identify a problem and then assist in the development of possible solutions. Alternatives may be developed through individual or organizational responses (see Chapters 4, 5, and 6). In either case, they are tailored for one person's specific needs.[9]

All the resources of the organization should be brought to bear to help a responder suffering from a stress-related incident. Special programs, including employee or volunteer assistance programs, personal counseling, communications skills training, problem-solving training, a buddy system, team building sessions, financial counseling, or other support services, should be utilized, if available (see Chapters 5 and 6).

Despite all interventions that might be applied, some responders will need more intensive psychological support. For these people there is an additional level of intervention, *referral*.

r
e
a
p
e
REFERRAL

For people who need professional intervention, referrals should be made as soon as possible. Referral does not mean that the system has failed or that it could not take care of its own. Just as any person has limits, so does an organization. It is acknowledgment of these limits that allows the system to reach beyond itself and incorporate associated mental health professionals as adjuncts.

Each organization should develop a list of professionals who have some experience in working with emergency personnel or a sincere willingness to assist them. The list should include those who are good educators and those who are able to provide effective services such as debriefings and counseling. Not every mental health professional is trained or interested in working with emergency personnel. Organizations should be cautious in selecting mental health professionals. Without the right orientation, training, and experience, they may be of little or no help and might even cause harm.[10]

SUMMARY

In this chapter we have presented a brief overview of the Reaper model for stress interventions in emergency services. It was developed to provide a systematic approach to establishing stress interventions for emergency personnel. It is not the only approach for stress reduction. It is simply one approach.

For a very long time emergency services personnel were ignored when it came to their psychological needs. It was always assumed that they were specially trained and immune to stress. That myth has forced many to keep silent about their needs even when this caused them great pain. Hopefully, this book has assisted in eliminating the myth that emergency people do not experience stress in their jobs. Perhaps it will serve as a starting point and guidebook for individuals and organizations that want to do something about emergency services stress.

For additional information on stress management training programs, contact either:

Jeffrey T. Mitchell, Ph.D.
Emergency Health Services Department
University of Maryland Baltimore County
5401 Wilkens Avenue
Baltimore, MD 21228
(301) 455-3223

or

Grady P. Bray, Ph.D., President
Human Potentials
1654 Monroe Avenue
Rochester, NY 14618
(716) 244-4969

REFERENCES

1. Robinson, R. (1986). *Health and Stress in Ambulance Services.* Melbourne, Australia: Social Biology Resources Centre.
2. Seyle, H. (1974). *Stress without Distress.* Philadelphia: J.B. Lippincott.
3. Seyle, H. (1956). *The Stress of Life.* New York: Free Press.
4. Hartsough, D. M., and Garaventa Myers, D. (1985). Effects of stress on disaster workers. In D. M. Hartsough and D. Garaventa Myers, Eds., *Disaster Work and Mental Health: Prevention and Control of Stress among Workers.* Rockville, MD: Center for Mental Health Studies of Emergencies, U.S. Department of Health and Human Services.
5. Harris, V. (1988). Coping with stress in the emergency services family. Presented Apr. 6, 1988 for the Howard County, Maryland Fire Department.
6. Mitchell, J. T. (1983). Guidelines for psychological debriefings. *Emergency Management Course Manual.* Emmitsburg, MD: Federal Emergency Management Agency, Emergency Management Institute.
7. Kennedy-Ewing, L. (1988). *Delaware County Critical Incident Stress Management Program.* Media, PA: Delaware County Department of Human Resources.
8. Cooper, C. (1981). *The Stress Check.* Englewood Cliffs, NJ: Spectrum Books.
9. Monat, A., and Lazarus, R. S. (Eds.). (1985). *Stress and Coping: An Anthology.* 2nd Ed. New York: Columbia University Press.
10. Duckworth, D. H. (1986). Psychological problems arising from disaster work. *Stress Medicine, 2:* 315–323.

APPENDIX:
STRESS MEASUREMENT SCALES

SCALE 1   Stress Fact or Fiction Quiz

How much do you know about stress? Answer the following statements to test your knowledge:

1. People who feel stress are nervous to start with. True or False?
2. You always know when you are under stress. True or False?
3. Prolonged physical exercise will weaken your resistance to stress. True or False?
4. Stress is always bad. True or False?
5. Stress can cause unpleasant problems, but at least it cannot kill you. True or False?
6. Stress can be controlled with medication. True or False?
7. Work-related stress can be left at the office and not brought home. True or False?
8. Stress is only in the mind; it is not physical. True or False?
9. Stress can be eliminated. True or False?
10. There is nothing you can do about stress without making drastic changes in your life-style. True or False?

The correct answer to all ten questions is *False.* If you answered *True* to even one, you are a victim of a stress myth.

Reprinted with permission of The Free Press, a Division of Macmillan, Inc. from *Managing Job Stress and Health: The Intelligent Person's Guide* by Michael T. Matteson and John M. Ivancevich. Copyright © 1982 by The Free Press.

SCALE 2   Tension Quotient Test

To test your tension quotient, respond to the statements below. Assign them a value from 1 to 5 based on how they most clearly relate to your behavior (1, Never; 2, Seldom; 3, Occasionally; 4, Frequently; 5, Always). When you are finished, add up your points and find where you fall on the risk scale.

Type A Personality

1. I am tense.

2. I am highly competitive.

3. I am plagued by deadlines.

4. I am subjected to many stressful events (home life, work, financial, etc.)

To Score:

    4–8: Little to no risk
  9–12: Low to moderate risk
13–16: Moderate to high risk
17–20: Potential problem or crisis

Anxiety

1. I feel anxious and tense.

2. I am afraid of such things as being alone, experiencing new things, and being in crowds or closed places.

3. I am restless, uneasy, and/or unable to relax.

4. I wake up too early and/or am unable to stay asleep.

Autonomy

1. I enjoy being unattached to people or things.

2. I resent people who try to regulate my conduct.

3. I could live in a very lonely place.

4. I would enjoy being my own boss, working alone.

5. I consider myself to be independent and free.

To Score:

  5–10: Little to no risk
11–15: Low to moderate risk
16–20: Moderate to high risk
21–25: Potential problem or crisis

Aggression

1. I do my best not to let people get the best of me.

2. I feel that certain people need to be put in "their place."

3. I let it be known when I am angry.

4. I get angry at myself and other people.

5. I have weak feelings and/or shakiness or dizzy spells.

5. I experience instant anger if things do not go as I had planned.

6. I let people know when they do something I do not like.

7. I tend to criticize others under any circumstances.

To Score:

 5–10: Little to no risk
11–15: Low to moderate risk
16–20: Moderate to high risk
21–25: Potential problem or crisis

To Score:

 7–14: Little to no risk
15–21: Low to moderate risk
22–28: Moderate to high risk
29–35: Potential problem or crisis

From W. D. Brown, *Welcome Stress! It Can Help You Be Your Best* (Minnesota: CompCare Publishers, 1983). Reprinted with permission from the author.

SCALE 3   Measuring Life Stress

Holmes and his colleagues (Holmes & Holmes, 1970; Holmes & Rahe, 1967; Rahe & Arthur, 1978) have developed a scale, the Social Readjustment Rating Scale, which reflects the cumulative stress to which an individual has been exposed over a period of time. "Life change units" are used to measure life stress in the following areas.

Events	Scale of Impact	Events	Scale of Impact
Death of spouse	100	Son or daughter leaving home	29
Divorce	73		
Marital separation	65	Change in responsibility at work	29
Jail term	63		
Death of close family member	63	Outstanding personal achievement	28
Personal injury or illness	53	Wife begins/stops work	26
Marriage	50	Begin or end school	26
Fired at work	47	Change in living conditions	25
Marital reconciliation	45		
Retirement	45	Revision of personal habits	24
Change in health of family member	44	Trouble with boss	23
Pregnancy	39	Change in work hours or conditions	20
Sex difficulties	39	Change in residence	20
Gain of new family member	39	Change in schools	20
Business readjustment	39	Change in recreation	19
Change in financial state	38	Change in church activity	19
Death of close friend	37	Change in social activity	18
Change to different line of work	36	Small mortgage or loan	17
		Change in sleep habits	16
Change in number of arguments with spouse	35	Change in number of family get-togethers	15
High mortgage	31	Change in eating habits	15
Foreclosure of mortgage or loan	30	Vacation	13
		Christmas	12
Trouble with in-laws	29	Minor violations of the law	11

For persons who had been exposed in recent months to stressful events that added up to an LCU score of 300 or above, these investigators found the risk of developing a major illness within the next two years to be very high, approximating 80 percent.

Holmes and Rahe, "Social Readjustment Rating Scale," *Journal of Psychosomatic Research,* Vol. 11, No. 2 (1967), 213–18. Reprinted with permission from Dr. Thomas H. Holmes and Pergamon Press.

SCALE 4   Type A Profile

Check all following self-descriptive statements:

_____ Speak the last few words of your sentence rapidly.

_____ Always move, walk, and eat rapidly.

_____ Feel impatient with the rate at which most events take place.

_____ Usually attempt to finish others' sentences.

_____ Become unduly irritated when traffic is slow.

_____ Find it intolerable to watch others do tasks you could do faster.

_____ Usually look for summaries of interesting literature.

_____ Indulge in polyphasic thought, trying to think of or do two or more things simultaneously.

_____ Ponder business problems while away from the office.

_____ Pretend to listen to others but remain preoccupied with your own thoughts.

_____ Almost always feel vaguely guilty when you relax.

_____ Do not take time to appreciate surroundings (i.e., sunsets, scenic beauty, etc.).

_____ Attempt to schedule more and more in less and less time.

_____ Possess a chronic sense of time urgency.

_____ Feel compelled to challenge another like yourself.

_____ Recognize aggressive behavior in yourself that may not be noticed by others.

_____ Frequently clench fist in conversation.

_____ Bang your hand on a table or pound one fist into palm of other to emphasize a point.

_____ Habitually clench your jaw or grind your teeth.

_____ Believe that your success has been due to your ability to get things done faster than others.

_____ Evaluate your own and others' activities in terms of numbers.

_____ Total

Key: Total the number of checks made above. If there are seven or fewer, there is little likelihood you are a Type A personality; seven to twelve checks indicates a tendency toward a Type A personality structure, while more than twelve suggests that you are a Type A personality.

SCALE 5   A Quiz on Job and Career Stressors

This is the third and final portion of the stress diagnostic survey. As previously, use the 1 to 7 rating scale for each item.

Stress Diagnostic Survey—
Job and Career Stressors

> Record a *1* if the condition is never a source of stress.
> *2* if the condition is rarely a source of stress.
> *3* if the condition is occasionally a source of stress.
> *4* if the condition is sometimes a source of stress.
> *5* if the condition is often a source of stress.
> *6* if the condition is usually a source of stress.
> *7* if the condition is always a source of stress.

Your rating

_____ 1. I work on many unnecessary job activities.

_____ 2. My job objectives are unclear to me.

_____ 3. To keep up with my job, I usually have to take work home with me.

_____ 4. My job is boring.

_____ 5. I am responsible for people.

_____ 6. My job pushes me hard to finish on time.

_____ 7. My work area (office, space) is too crowded.

_____ 8. I do not have enough opportunities to advance in this organization.

_____ 9. I have job activities that are accepted by one person and not by others.

_____ 10. I do not have the authority to do my job well.

_____ 11. My job is too difficult.

_____ 12. My job has become too routine.

_____ 13. I must make decisions that affect the career, safety, or lives of other people.

_____ 14. There is not enough time in the day to do my job.

_____ 15. Work conditions on my job are below par.

_____ 16. I am at a standstill in my career.

_____ 17. I receive conflicting requests from two or more people.

_____ 18. I am not sure what is expected of me.

_____ 19. I am responsible for too many jobs.

_____ **20.** My job is too easy.

_____ **21.** I am responsible for helping others solve their problems.

_____ **22.** I do not have time to take an occasional break from the job.

_____ **23.** My working conditions are not as good as the working conditions of others.

_____ **24.** I am in a career that offers little promise for the future.

Reprinted with permission of The Free Press, a Division of Macmillan, Inc. from *Managing Job Stress and Health: The Intelligent Person's Guide* by Michael T. Matteson and John M. Ivancevich. Copyright © 1982 by The Free Press.

SCALE 6   Level of Marital Satisfaction

Answer each of the following items True or False as you assess your marriage at present:

True	False	
_____	_____	1. My marriage is as fulfilling as I had expected.
_____	_____	2. The times I am glad I am married far outnumber those when I wish I were still single.
_____	_____	3. My mate is generally respectful of my feelings.
_____	_____	4. I am usually considerate of my mate's desires.
_____	_____	5. Most of my daydreams and fantasies involve my mate in a complimentary manner.
_____	_____	6. When I have a free evening, I prefer spending it with my mate.
_____	_____	7. Both of us are increasingly finding areas of agreement the longer we are married.
_____	_____	8. Our philosophies on handling money, relating to in-laws, and socializing with friends are similar.
_____	_____	9. Each of us has individual friends, as well as couple friends both of us enjoy.
_____	_____	10. I feel assured that I can trust my mate with *any* secret, knowing my trust would never be betrayed.

Key: Eight or more True answers indicates a strong, healthy marriage. Five to seven True answers suggest a basically healthy marriage, but one that could benefit from working together in areas answered in the negative. Four or fewer True answers place a marriage in a category of possible jeopardy. Help would probably be beneficial from some professional affiliated with the American Association of Marriage and Family Therapists, an organization of professionals who by their training are especially equipped to help couples work through marital and family problems.

From W. D. Brown, Welcome Stress! It Can Help You Be Your Best (Minnesota: CompCare Publishers, 1983). Reprinted with permission.

SCALE 7   Signs of Stress

Do you recognize signs of stress when they occur? Awareness of these signs can help you recognize stress early, channeling it into eustress rather than distress. Remember: *you are not trying to eliminate stress but to direct it so that most of your stress will not lead to distress.*

Carefully read the following behaviors and physical reactions, putting a "1" in front of the ones that *nearly always* accompany stress for you. Then read the list again, rating with a "2" those which *sometimes* occur with your stress. Finally, record a "3" beside those which happen *infrequently.*

_____ Depression	_____ Rapid pulse rate
_____ Withdrawal	_____ Increased perspiration
_____ Hyperactivity	_____ Pounding heart
_____ Compulsiveness	_____ Tightened stomach
_____ Muscle tension	_____ Appetite loss
_____ Shortness of breath	_____ Overeating
_____ Gritting teeth	_____ Sleeping more frequently or longer than usual
_____ Biting lips	
_____ Disrupted sleep patterns	_____ Clenching jaw
_____ Excessive emotional display	_____ Racing thoughts

Study your own ratings. Often, just recognizing how you react in certain situations will give you the opportunity to improve or even eliminate the negative effects of stress. Pay particular attention to those you have rated a "1." Are there ways you can rechannel your energy, avoiding the most troublesome symptoms of stress?

From W. D. Brown, Welcome Stress! It Can Help You Be Your Best (Minnesota: CompCare Publishers, 1983). Reprinted with permission.

SCALE 8   Symptoms of Stress

Check each of the following which you experience with some degree of frequency.

_____ Fatigue	A depressed person tires easily. Previous levels of energy may have diminished appreciably.
_____ Insomnia	While sleep may be intensely desired, it is elusive once the person has retired for the evening. A similar condition is noted when one regularly awakens early with feelings of exhaustion or fright.
_____ Inability to concentrate	After watching a television program, listening to a lecture, or even participating in a conversation, little content can be recalled.
_____ Remorse	Guilt is frequently noted in the depressed person, arising over either acts of commission or omission.
_____ Indecision	Many depressed people cannot make up their minds about anything. Even the simplest decisions seem too difficult for them.
_____ Decreased affection	It may come as a surprise, but the depressed person may feel little affection toward those much loved in the past.
_____ Reduced sexual interest	The depressed individual may have little interest in participating in sexual relations.
_____ Anxiety	Depression may be accompanied by feelings of tension, anxiety, or fright. Sometimes these feelings are so strong that they mask their underlying cause—depression.

_____ Irritability	The depressed person is easily annoyed and impatient, particularly over trivial things.
_____ Thoughts of suicide	Occasional thoughts of suicide are not uncommon in the depressed person. Fortunately, these ideas disappear when the person starts to feel better, but if they persist, indicate a need for immediate professional help.
_____ Concern about dying	Hardly a paradox following the mention of suicide, fearfulness of imminent death may be another symptom of depression. In actuality, a concern with both suicide and dying are frequently noted in the same depressed person.

Note: Rating depression with a numerical scale suggests but does not diagnose the seriousness of the problem. In general, five or fewer checks indicate mild depression; six or seven moderate, and eight or more serious depression. Of course, a seriously depressed person needs professional help. However, any person who feels that his or her depression is not manageable or is out of control should consult a therapist for treatment and/or referral.

From W. D. Brown, *Welcome Stress! It Can Help You Be Your Best* (Minnesota: CompCare Publishers, 1983). Reprinted with permission.

INDEX